I0478879

It's Time For The Ultimate Cure

From the Real Poisoning of America

By

Roy Knight Jr

Damaged and Concerned Consumer

ISBN:**13: 9781540421029**

ISBN:**10:1540421023**

ACKNOWLEDGMENTS

This would not have been possible without the research and instruction given by Dr. David Perlmutter and Dr. William Davis and Dr. Daniel Amen. The British Medical Journal, the New England Journal of Medicine, NIH's PubMed and Wikipedia also were very important in the construction of this book. I tried to attribute every passage used from these sources.

Credit also goes to James, for without his comments," No one even knows or cares about this".
Photos By:
© Nui7711 | Dreamstime.com - **Stethoscope, medicine capsules and banknotes**
© Jevtic | Dreamstime.com - **Business partners on wheat field**
© Walter Arce | Dreamstime.com - **Yellow Crop Duster**
© Wolfberry | Dreamstime.com - **Health Risks of Obesity**
© Pratin Charnnarong | Dreamstime.com - **Pill**
IMAGE COURTESY OF AREEYA AT FREEDIGITALPHOTOS.NET
© Wolfberry | Dreamstime.com

© Arrow | Dreamstime.com - **Brain and solution**

I followed *It's Time for a Cure* with The Ultimate Cure because the first book didn't tell the whole story. Although that book doesn't complete the story, its importance is as crucial to know. The information in my first book, *It's Time For a Cure,* details 17 disorders and diseases and how they're influenced by glycation which is influenced by glucose consumption. Honestly, that was all I thought this was responsible for. Then, I looked into it deeper, and the deeper I delved into it, the bleaker the picture got. Then all of a sudden it turned ugly, really ugly.

This has now become a movement. This is a movement to bring back sanity and dignity to America and the world. That sanity and dignity have been stolen from us for the last thirty years. It goes back to the time when a company started dabbling in genetically modified seeds and soon earned a patent for a creation of nature, a seed. This is a story of a for-profit chemical corporation and their political engineering of our government, to assume control over government agencies, and the desire of that corporation to completely control our food supply. With the help of some strategic placements in the Supreme Court and certain gov't agencies, this corporation has succeeded in acquiring unprecedented control over the food we eat and what that creates. What it creates in itself, is devastating. The only way to stop the destruction that this industry is responsible for is to stop buying their products until they decide to change them and give us something healthier to eat. That's the reason for this book series. *It's Time For A Cure!* The world must know what is being done to them without their consent or knowledge

Part I

Dependence

(The Addiction)

Chapter 1

Confessions of a Reformed Carboholic

Sugar, I love it. I grew up loving it. Because I grew up loving it, I'm now addicted to it. It's an addiction that was forced upon me by our food industry, telling my mother that she had to make refined and whole grains the most prevalent food in my diet. She fed me this food, supposedly, to keep me healthy. Aren't whole grains supposed to make you healthy? That was 60 years ago. I'm paying the price for that now, with my arthritis. I was paying the price for it just 30 months ago, by carrying 30 lbs more than what I carry right now and being borderline diabetic and in pain all the time. I'm about to debunk this myth that whole grains are healthy. There is a price to be paid for eating a (starchy) carbohydrate diet and you're paying it with every sandwich you eat, every corn chip you munch, and every noodle you eat.

My sisters are paying the price for it now, also. They are both obese and diabetic. My father has always exercised to keep his weight down. He's always been able to burn off the excess glucose until he was about 35. Even though he's always jogged every day, since I was in 7th grade, he couldn't run away from this. After being borderline diabetic he couldn't change his downhill spiral. He's now taking an anti-diabetes drug which has several side effects that are initially so small that they aren't noticed but after time, start to inflict other harm to the body, due to the effects of the chemical changes caused by medication. His carb diet is starting to lead him down the same path as my mother, who passed away 4 months ago. My mother, in trying to be the best mother and wife she could be, went along with what the FDA and the USDA told her because she wanted to do what was right for her family. Guidelines from the USDA telling her that grains needed to be at the base of her all of her meals was what drove her to do this to our family. This is what doomed us to our current list of ailments, ailments like obesity and diabetes, arthritis, cancer, stomach ailments galore, and now, side effects from treatment for those ailments. It all comes along with a carbohydrate diet because all carbs break down into glucose. Even yet, *MyPlate.gov* suggests that whole grains be a part of a healthy diet. The evidence I'm going to show you is completely contrary to this notion.

Because sugar addiction is America's biggest addiction, that makes it, its worst addiction. It's an addiction that everybody grew up with and into. It's an addiction that's been with us for as long as we've been eating it. It's an addiction that's become far worse than it's ever been since we've been eating it over its 10,000-year history. It's an addiction that's built scores of empires, and then tore them all down. This addiction is far worse than any other addiction that plagues America. Whether it be today, yesterday or tomorrow, this addiction is the worst that Man has ever faced or may ever face. This is simply due to its propensity to expand its influence across the whole world. It's also driven by the greed of those condemned to this addiction. Their desire to feed their own addiction drives them to impose this addiction on the rest of the world, simply so they can make an extra buck. This addiction is at the root of almost every known form of dementia, heart disease, diabetes and everything that comes along with that, like cancers, cardiovascular diseases. The list is endless because sugar's worst instigator of inflammation, AGEs, or glycation is at the base of an arm-long list of disorders.

All of these disorders can be curbed simply by curbing carbohydrate consumption but addiction keeps this from happening. That's why fighting this addiction, in particular, is so important. It's life-saving at its simplest, just remove contaminating factors from the food source and the diseases cannot manifest themselves. The contaminating factor in this case? You guessed it, sugar. Sugar addiction is leading our society to the brink of destruction because of the nature of its addiction and what it does to the body. Its continued use only leads to discomfort and death. It's only redeeming factor is that it tastes good and satiates quickly. This is what makes it so deadly, though.

That's sad. I have to live with it too. I can't have what I love, what I've been addicted to. I have to say no, to stay healthy. So do you. I know that's exactly the opposite of what you've been told, but what you were told is wrong. For us, it's dead wrong. It should have never been pushed upon us to eat it in the quantities that it was. But pushed upon us it was. And we bought it. We bought into it big time and we're paying for it now. This is evidenced by the proliferation of Alzheimer's disease. How many lives does it have to take, before people wake up? How many families does it have to destroy, before people wake up?

Carbolism Should Be Treated Like Alcoholism

We need clinics for sugar addiction and they should be financed by the food industrial complex that imposed this diet on the people who now suffer the consequences of it. The administration of the clinic though should be done by trained medical professionals, because this is an addiction and should be treated as such.

Is this something that should be investigated? Should an industry be held accountable for the ruse that's been pulled on the American people, and now the world? The ruse is that this is healthy food when it's really not. Why are they still allowed to claim that it's healthy? Why are they still, allowed to advertise that it's healthy? It's clearly not, and it's clearly at the root of almost all of the deadliest diseases, that we're actively fighting right now. Diseases like Atherosclerosis, Endocarditis, and Hypertensive heart disease. That's just the CVD's. We haven't even covered the cancers or dementias. Those lists are much longer. Can anyone tell me why this is still allowed to be advertised like it is today?

It starts with what's put in baby food for starches and fillers and sweeteners. These fillers satiate babies quickly often putting them right to sleep after a short burst of energy. This is the first indication of sugar addiction and it starts at a young age. This is done for a purpose. That purpose is to addict you to its lure, so you'll buy into it when you're an adult. It continues with your introduction to breakfast cereals and the load of sugars they carry when you see them advertised with the Saturday morning cartoons. I can remember commercials for Sugar Pops, Sugar Frosted Flakes, and Captain Crunch. I can remember how I used to beg my mother for these foods. It starts young, real young and continues through your youth with candy and soda, and into your adult years with bread, corn chips, oatmeal, and pasta.

It's been forced upon us. Nobody has had a choice in this addiction and that is what makes it so lethal. That also makes it profitable for the Pharmaceutical industry. This is what scares me. The Pharmaceutical industry used to be owned by the same industry the provided the crop seed for the farmers that grew the grain that provided the flour to bake all of those loaves of bread that cause so much disease.

The Perfect Ruse

It's almost the perfect scam. Sell crop seed to farmers that have been genetically modified, so that it feeds your customer base, food that will require them, in the future to purchase medications from your other companies. How convenient we've made it for this industry to take our money. We should be ashamed.

We would be ashamed if we knew that this was done intentionally, especially if it was done for nothing more than profit. That is why this is something that should be investigated. Regardless of how long it takes, we need to know who is responsible. This is a lesson that cannot be lost, like every other study done on these concerns; we cannot allow this to be swept under the rug. Even if they're no longer around, we need to hold their companies' accountable. This is the only way we can prevent this from happening in the future.

For 1,000s of years, we've been treating the symptoms of the diseases and disorders that carbohydrate digestion cause. Because of our addiction to it, we've never looked at the prospect of eliminating the cause completely. When a whole society is addicted to a staple that they've eaten their whole lives, how does one tell the truth about something that is so important to everyone on the planet? How does one tell everyone that what they're eating is killing them slowly, expensively, painfully, and worst of all, undignified because of all the lost memories of brain damage? How does one tell a whole society that a staple that they've lived on for close to 10,000 years has been, and continues to be, the one food that creates more disease and illness than any other one food in their diet? How does a world break their addiction, when the addicted are the majority of the world and only 5% of that population can recognize their addiction?

Dr. Perlmutter is trying to tell the people and continues to do so. I honestly feel that he thinks as I do, that if we don't dispel the consumption of these foods, our society is doomed. From what I've learned since I've broken the addiction, I see a collapse, due to out of control emotions, due to the wild glucose swings in the blood, making people under the control of a carbohydrate diet, under the control of those who impose this diet on the American public. It's in their interest to keep America addicted and the best way they can do this is to tell you that it's healthy and what you need to keep your body healthy. Only those who want to buy their pharmaceuticals, from them in the future, are ones who should buy their food products now, because, they eventually will.

By following what little advice I offer, to curb your carbs dramatically and as completely as possible, you can dramatically slow down if not eliminate many of the disorders and diseases within these pages. If it can't eliminate your disease, it will reduce the expression of your disorder. If it doesn't cure you, it will definitely extend your life. My goal is to extend it a minimum of 20 years. I would like to see everyone live to be 100 years old, or more. I know this ~~diet~~ lifestyle can do that (depending on your age and degree of addiction of course). To know this yourself, though, you have to change your diet.

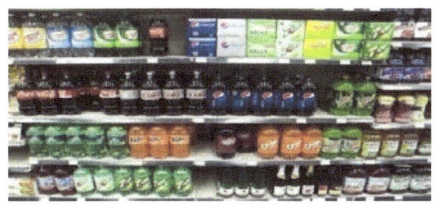

A Display of Dependence You Don't Need

Chapter 2
BREAD – THE STAFF OF DEATH

I know that bread is supposed to be the staff of life. I know that's what the Bible tells us. So does the Torah, and the Quran. That's because these groups of people have been eating this substance longer than anyone else in the world. Wheat has long been a staple for western Asians and Europeans and now, Americans. It's grown out of our cradle of civilization and we've grown addicted to it right out of our cradles.

Bread has been with us for more than our lifetimes and that is what makes it so dangerous, now. Because we all grew up with it, we've been addicted to it all of our lives, making it more difficult to break from, than any other addiction. Because it's such an integral part of our society, that makes it even harder to conquer.

But conquer it we must if we're to save our society from all of the illness and disease we're fighting right now and advance to the stars and find other planets to live on. We all know that this planet is getting too small for our expanding population and if we're to survive as a species, we need to find alternatives for everything destructive that we have allowed to creep into our lives.

Unfortunately, that includes bread, the staff of life. What used to be the staff of life is now the staff of death. This is mostly due to the genetic modifying that has taken place in our growing fields. With the introduction of GMO crop seed, it's changed the face of our diet, worldwide. Even though these new crops are able to feed millions of more people, they're doing it, at what cost? Of the millions of people it's feeding, it's them feeding them disease and death, due to the massive amount of glucose being introduced into everybody who eats it. This glucose is basically glue. That's what gluten means in Latin and it's this stuff that is gumming up everyone's body that eats this glue. Gluten, after all, is the basis of most grains. In wheat, it's particularly bad, because of its contents are of amylose and amylopectin, the foundation of amyloid plaque, which is the foundation of more disease than any other kind of plaque.

What started out as a way to feed the masses and try to stave off starvation, became deadlier than 5 nuclear bombs. People every, are dying from digesting this food. But, that's not the saddest part of this story. Everyone dying is dying without any dignity because of what this food does to your brain. It eats it up and there's nothing you can do about it unless you shut it off at the spigot.

Bread eats up your brain in multiple ways, starting with the gliadin in gluten. Gliadin has the ability to make your body send out anti-gliadin antibodies which have the ability to eat up brain cells in your cerebellum. That spells brain damage and there's nothing you can do about it if you eat bread. The more bread you eat, the more brain you lose. It's that simple. I'm sorry, but that's the story. You can't change it unless you stop the consumption of it.

Bread has always had a capability to do this, just not to the extent, it does so today. Bread has always eaten up our brains, but past varieties of wheat were not nearly as destructive as they are today, with the emergence of GMOs.

This is what makes bread so dangerous today. The high glucose content of bread not only feeds your brain these anti-gliadin antibodies, the amylose and amylopectin found in the gluten of wheat, contribute to amyloid plaque, which is the foundation of more illnesses and diseases than any other single substance we electively put in our bodies (even cigarette smoke).

Dependence Courtesy of Monsanto's Crop Seed Industry

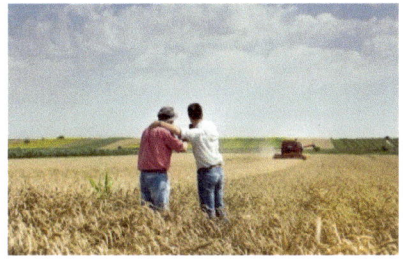

Even though this addiction has been with us since the dawn of civilization, the industry responsible for putting it on our tables to eat, in trying to make a buck, has inadvertently addicted our entire society to this substance, in a worse manner than our species has ever experienced before. This affects our entire society, as it has given us a worse addiction to fight. Fight if you must, though. If you don't fight it, a world of hurt lies directly in your path.

The world of hurt includes a multitude of cardiovascular diseases, most cancers, almost all digestive disorders, 98% all brain disorders, and continued addiction to keep feeding these diseases. This, in my opinion, is the biggest and worst crime ever committed on the American public and the world. It has to stop and the quicker it happens, the better for our society.

I mentioned above that we need to conquer it to go to the stars. You're probably wondering why I mentioned this. (Bravo to those who already know.) We cannot go to the stars on a carbohydrate diet. A carb diet requires too much food to sustain it, to give us the ability to exist in space where we won't be able to grow food for centuries to come. That means that we need another food source other than carbs and guess what? Using fat in the diet to sustain us, is the only way our species will thrive in the stars. Here's the key, our diet must not rely on carbs in space. It just requires too much food to be sustainable. Carbs require you to replenish your reserves every couple hours or so and that kind of sustenance will not work in space. We'll be required to go longer lengths of time between meals and that means we must make every meal last that much longer if we're to travel to the stars. To me it's simple.

Being on an MTC ketogenic diet myself, I now know the diet, that will sustain us in our travels to the stars and it's not a carbohydrate diet. If' we remain resigned to our carbohydrate diet, we'll also have to take massive amounts of medications to the stars with us to combat all the disorders and diseases that these carbs are responsible for. That to me is not sustainable. Medications always bring with them, side effects. Medications don't usually cure a disease as much as they just make the symptoms of the disease tolerable. In space, we'll require the ability to cure diseases, not just treat them. Treatment is only for those who wish to continue taking medications. That is totally unsustainable in space.

I'm working on a complete chapter or even section on our travels to the stars and our need for a different diet to do so. Look for it in *Cure for the World*.

If we're to move to the stars, we have to do it without a carbohydrate diet. It's that simple. To me, it is time for a cure and you can't find it with medication. The only way it can only be done, is through diet. Just say no to glucose. Just say no to bread, what used to be our staff of life, has become our staff of death.

It's become apparent to me that our society is more concerned with profits than they are with health. This love affair with profits is what's costing our society it's health as a society and costing everyone within our society, dearly....quite often to the point of sacrificing lives for the sake of addiction and profits.

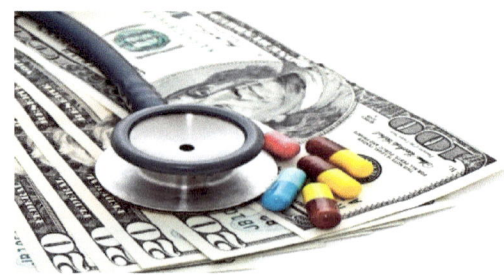

CHAPTER 3

Our Celebration of Our Addiction to Sugar and the Price We Pay For It.

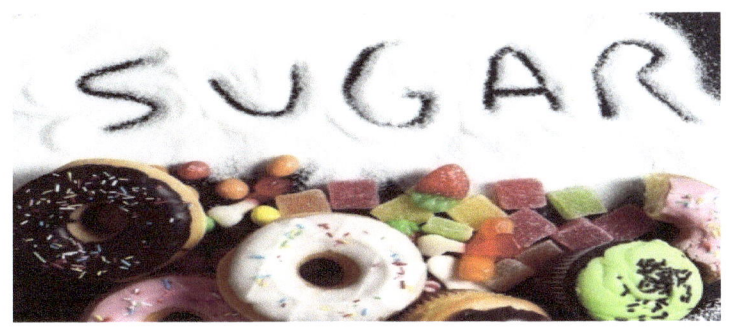

It's not hard to see how much you enjoy celebrating your addiction to carbs. It's displayed in everything that's said and done, in all aspects of the food industry. It's boldly advertised everywhere you go. Soon after following this celebration of addiction that you love to express, comes a parade of drugs that you'll be taking to treat all of the symptoms that come from succumbing to your addiction. This simple equation displays the need that we have to curb the influence of the grain and pharmaceutical industry on our health.

Failure to control this influence will not only lead to more disease and illness but more so, to greater health costs overall. How are we ever going to learn to live healthily and kick this habit, before it destroys our society? How are we ever going to put an end to diabetes? Or an end to Alzheimer's disease? Or cancer? Or heart disease? Or arthritis? Or hypertension? Hyperlipidemia? High Cholesterol? I would like to show just how our celebration of addiction to sugar is not only destroying our individual lives, it has the potential of destroying our entire civilization, if we don't curb is an influence.

I intend to show you how this industry hooks you in the first place, how they keep you hooked so in the future you're forced to buy into their drug habit. This drug habit involves NSAIDS (aspirin, Motrin, Advil, Aleve), anti-inflammatories, antacids, anti-gas and bloating, (Pepto Bismol, Gaviscon, Alka Seltzer) and we're just starting with the OCDs. For prescription medicine, we're looking at all opioids (Oxycontin, Oxycodone, Vicodin, Percocet), which again are addictive. More prescription NSAIDS like Celebrex, Relafen, Relifex, and Gambaran. We know that by the existing opioid abuse epidemic how dangerous these drugs are. Do you think this happened by chance?

Other prescription medicines that you're doomed to need if you continue your carbohydrate consumption (especially for those who allow ECC to control them), includes but are not limited to statins, vasoactive agents, fibrates, CETP Inhibitors, and niacin, just for starters. Statins are, by far, the far worst of these medications.

After spending 15 years giving care to and for seniors, I have seen the ravages statin drugs have taken on their bodies. They slowly rob their users from their mental faculties, then their muscles, then their lives. What it takes away from its users is in no way replaced by the treatment it offers. They are nothing more than invitations to a need to take more and more drugs. It seems that the drug industry has found ways to make you buy more of their wares.

Cholesterol, your body's fuel

This industry promotes that high cholesterol has something to do with heart disease, which couldn't be further from the truth and that high cholesterol is dangerous. This was first disputed close to 70 years ago. Cholesterol isn't the problem. Cholesterol is healthy. Your body has to use it to stay alive. Taking cholesterol away from your body only leads to more medication. I can see where this would benefit the drug industry.

High cholesterol isn't a heart problem. It's a diet problem. Your diet is responsible for your high cholesterol. Your major food source is your primary source of cholesterol and that is where the problem begins. Your high carbohydrate diet produces cholesterol in your body that is not clean cholesterol, meaning that it is dirty fuel, as cholesterol is your body's fuel. This is cholesterol you don't need. You need clean cholesterol that's been produced by fat. That is what powers our bodies.

Cholesterol is your body's fuel source. It's cholesterol that enters the cell to be used for fuel, so what's important is the kind of cholesterol that your body uses. Is it clean or dirty cholesterol? Cholesterol from carbohydrates is a dirty sticky fuel due to nature of which this cholesterol comes from. It comes from a sticky, icky, gooey, gluey substance, sugar or glucose and because of that, it has glycating effects on your body. This is what leads to plaque, the basis of almost all cancers, heart diseases and all dementias.

I've only talked about heart medications so far, I haven't even touched on cancer medication or cholesterol medication (many of which are related to heart medications like statins), nor have I covered other prescription medication for arthritis, high blood pressure, and memory loss. The list goes on and on. What a quagmire this has turned out to be. But I'm going to try to make some sense out of this quagmire, so that we're left with just a small puzzle leaving you wondering, like me, why?

I've already proven how the discontinuance of these foods leads only to better health and how continued consumption of these foods, only leads to a path of illness and disease. What I don't know, did this industry know what these foods do from the studies that have come out over the last 70+ years? Or did they remain electively ignorant of the reports? Or did they influence the cover-up of these reports? With as many reports that have come out, I seriously doubt it. There are just so many of them (701) that it's easy to miss most of them. Later I'll show you how this industry has had its problems in the courts. Some of it is not pretty.

I'll list just a few of the studies that have shown this damage going back over 70 years. The earliest study I found in 701 studies done over the years, was completed in 1939. I looked through page after page of studies that started in the 60's, 70's & the 80's. They seem to grow in number as time goes on. Studies have exploded since the turn of this century, as more and more people are starting to recognize the true dangers this food imposes on its consumers. Yet the majority of the addicted choose to remain ignorant to it dangers, as they're impotent in ignoring its lures. They are all controlled by their hormones which are controlling their emotions. This is a common trait of carbolism. The addicted have little to no choice in the matter. The need to feed the addiction is no less than that of any other addiction, which forces the addict to continue to feed the addiction. It's the way addiction works, it's the way carbolism works.

Celebration of sugar addiction

We're inundated with the commercialism of addiction on a daily basis. You see advertising for these foods and drinks everywhere. How many snack food companies are there? How many cereal companies are there? How many soft drink companies are there? How many beer and spirits companies are there? How many commercials do you see each day from these industries? All of those commercials are luring you into their web of addiction. The grain industry has found ways to infect our society, like seasonal flu or common cold affects all those who eat these grains. (And you thought your cold was just haphazard, something that you caught from someone else.)

We all know who profits from this today (Kraft, Nabisco, and Frito-Lay). But have you ever connected that with who is going to profit from it 10, 20, 30 years from now, the pharmaceutical industry? It seems that the grain industry's intent is to do nothing more than to fuel the drug industry. Whether it is their intent or not, it has been and is going to be, the end result. How long it continues to be, depends on how long you continue to allow your addictions to exist.

Drug companies, right now, are foaming at the mouth for all the business the food industry is sending them. (Pun intended.) Nobody is interested in breaking this addiction. What more could they ask for, a captive audience, all set up to need what they have an offer, to stop the pain, from the damage of their addiction at a cost that they set. You get to pay it or deal with your pain. Many times you have to pay it, just to stay alive. Do you wonder why medical costs keep going up or why insurance costs so much? The demand is so extensive, due to the addiction rate. Costs always rise when the demand for anything goes up.

If everyone would stop buying into this ruse, and find their cure, what would happen to the pharmaceutical industry? A huge drop in demand for their drugs would lower the price for the drugs as well as bring down the number of treatments, as well. What would happen to the medical industry if nobody needed it except for emergency treatment for injuries? What if the need to treat disease diminished to nothing? It's not hard to see the impact that would have. What would be the cost of keeping people alive and healthier longer? What if you could allow more people to be more active longer? What if no-one needed medication anymore?

The underlying cause of sugar addiction

First off, let's define it. Dictionary.com defines addiction; *Noun, the state of being enslaved to a habit or practice or to something that is psychologically or physically habit-forming, as narcotics, to such an extent that its cessation causes severe trauma.-*

Wikipedia definition; *"Addiction is a medical condition characterized by compulsive engagement in rewarding stimuli, despite adverse consequences."*

I personally define addiction as a compulsion to consume a substance that the body craves but doesn't need because it actually harms the body. This definition rings true for heroin and opioids, sugar and alcohol, cigarettes and tobacco, the three most abused substances in the civilized algorithm, although not in that order. The worst of these addictions is that of sugar and alcohol, with sugar being by far, the meanest and vilest scourge ever committed upon the human race.

It starts with the placement of sugar and carbs in the baby food that's sold throughout the industry. It's obvious to me why they put it in baby food. That's because it's so palatable and goes down so easy making the food more palatable so babies would be less likely to not consume it. What baby doesn't love the taste of sugar? This taste for sugar soon turns into an addiction requiring it be fed to the body, every other hour or so. Whether or not this was the intended consequences of the marketing of this food, this consequence has become America's newest death sentence. By showing how this addiction affects the body in *Carbs; The Newly Discovered Death*

Sentence, the evidence proves how dangerous this food is to human physiology. Yet we continue to celebrate our addiction to it simply to enhance profits. Profits for the Grain industry as well as the drug industry are driven by our insatiable appetites for these foods, which is driven by their unending advertising.

The major reason this addiction continues is due to the manner in which it is and has been promoted. The desire to create more and more ways and forms to entice everyone to eat and drink more of this deadly food is nothing short of astounding. It continues to amaze me how inventive we are at finding ways to kill ourselves with our own taste buds. Studies have been done, books have been written, the public has been warned, but it continues to happen. Every time I turn around I see another new way to kill ourselves in another appealing commercial. All this advertising encouraging us to consume more and more or their blood glucose raising, diabetes causing, HBP causing, dementia-causing foods is the driving force of this addiction and consequent expense. A carbohydrate diet requires that you feed it almost on an hourly basis.

A ketogenic diet, on the other hand, allows you to go all day without eating much of anything. Here's the secret, carboholics don't like to go hungry. They'll do almost anything they can to not go hungry. Those on a ketogenic diet don't mind going hungry. Actually, to us, it's not going hungry. It's simply going without eating. The hunger doesn't exist much, after the cycle of addiction has been broken. We feel the hunger pangs and many times, welcome them because we know that is where we build our better health. We do this by building Ghrelin throughout our systems because we know that Ghrelin works to build our immunity as well as making us a little smarter by increasing our brain power, through the addition of BDNF in our brains. Remember BDNF is that stuff that's the foundation of new brain cells. Remember the Nrf2, that ramps up the production of your anti-oxidants? Those are both benefits of Ghrelin in your system.

Your celebration of your addiction to this sugar is the industry's celebration of profits, both in the food, they sell us and the drugs we buy to relieve the pain. For them, it's a win-win situation. For the public who buys into this, it's a no-win situation. This is the prescription for future medications if you're in your teens and twenties. In your thirties, you'll start buying their headache and stomach ache medication. In your forties, it'll become insulin or anti-diabetes medication, then in your 50's and 60's and beyond, pick your poison, heart disease, cancer, Alzheimer's disease. Anyone or all of these are going to hit you when you least expect it. I know. I've experienced it. I pray that you heed my words and don't experience it yourselves.

Targeted Advertising

Almost everything I see advertised on channels marketing to younger viewers is encouraging everyone to buy more soda, energy drinks (most of which are laden with sugar), snack chips and cereals. Then when you're a few years older the ads are aimed at selling you crackers and pasta. Then into your 40's, 50's and 60's the ads are all aimed at selling you treatments and drugs for all the diseases and illnesses that your lifetime of consumption has brought you, drugs for diabetes, heart disease, cancer, arthritis, dementia, HBP, high cholesterol, etc, etc, etc. How long do I need to go on? Did I mention headaches or stomach aches?

When I watch programming on TV appealing to older viewers, like news broadcasts, I'm inundated with the commercials they show for drugs to treat heart disease (for there is no cure, only treatment), to treat cancer (again no cure), diabetes, high cholesterol, high blood pressure, arthritis, diabetes, and obesity. Drug companies are doing their best to sell their drugs to us to treat (not cure) us, for the illness and pain that they cause. And we buy it. We buy into it big time. We've bought into it our entire lives. The biggest problem here is most people are still buying into it. And they're buying into it in massive quantities, evidenced by pandemics of obesity, diabetes, Alzheimer's disease, heart disease, cancer, arthritis, HBP, etc, etc. What's being spent now, not just on snacks and beverages, but on staples like flour and sugar, pasta and cereal will be tripled, quadrupled, quintupled and even more, in payments to the pharmaceutical companies in the future, after your done paying the price for the damage all your years of consumption will cause. The only way to getting as close to a cure as you can is to give them up as completely as possible, otherwise, a continuance will only incur the need for drugs.

The drugs they'll be pushing on you, for heart disease or cancer, or even just for your headaches and stomach aches will be an array of SIDE EFFECT causing chemicals that will ultimately make it necessary for you to purchase more of their drugs to counteract the side effects of the drugs you've been taking for your treatment. You see proof of this everywhere. I experienced it myself when I was on 12 different medications just to treat an underlying chronic pain problem. I had to take diuretics for my high blood pressure, anti-depressants because "they worked on the same receptors in the brain that the pain used", NSAIDS for the headaches I always used to get, opioids for the chronic pain I live with from the car accident. The diuretics were for my high blood pressure caused by my pain, or so I thought. After I quit the bread, the pain subsided. Maybe not completely, but it to encouraged me enough to quit all grains. When it subsided, even more, I decided to quit all carbs. My biggest benefits were the loss of my high blood pressure along with 30 lbs of weight and the disappearance of the worst of my pain.

When they advertise new drugs, the precautions and side effects of the drugs they want to sell you, take up more of the commercials, they show, than the explanations of their benefits. I have to wonder where the regulation is. Is it for the consumer (which it's supposed to be) or is this regulation for the benefit of the industry? How can drugs with that many precautions and side effects still be approved for sale? It appears to me that this industry has the FDA under their spell.

Which does it appear to be, to you? This industry is still allowed to market foods of disease and death while marketing treatments for those diseases and illnesses. Who knew that these industries are related? Before I started this, I didn't. I had to uncover this information, so I'll show you how all of this is connected and it's connected to take your money. Their manner of taking your money is clearly hazardous to your health. This is something you need to know because nothing is more important than your health.

The Industry that Feeds you Sugar and Grains, Force you to Buy Drugs from their Pharmaceutical Industry

The food industry which also includes the grain industry, which includes the crop seed industry that provides the farmers with the seed they need to grow the grains that they sell us to put on our tables for us to eat, is related to the pharmaceutical industry that makes all the drugs for all the diseases that these foods create. My question is how could we allow an industry responsible for our food, be also responsible to treat the diseases their food creates? (This is the worst kind of *catch 22* for the consumer.)

What we've allowed these related industries to do, in a nutshell, is drain our wallets at the grocery store by influencing us to buy their sodas, fruit drinks, snack foods, corn chips, pastas, breads, cereals and crackers, while draining our wallets again at the pharmacy to buy their drugs that treat the symptoms of the diseases their food is responsible for. We pay three times;

1. For the food, we're sold through their marketing....(and their advertising is pure magic to see and it's so easy to buy into). Their product tastes better than anything in the world. How much more could you can ask for than a worldwide customer base that's addicted to your wares? Because it's addictive (like tobacco), you only have to make it more appealing than that of its competitors, of which it has plenty because the addiction is so strong. That makes it more deadly than heroin, simply because it's as prevalent as water. In some places, more prevalent.
2. We also get to pay their associates for the drugs we need to combat the diseases that their food has given us. And pay them we do. We'll pay them anything to get out of the pain that we've been inflicted with, from eating the food they so happily sold to us. We just don't connect that pain we feel with the food we've grown up with. But it is connected. It's

connected in a big way. They first connected themselves toward the end of the 20th century with mergers and acquisitions bringing chemical, pharmaceutical, and crop seed companies under one roof.

3. The largest price we pay is detailed in the next section, *The Damage*. I cover it extensively in chapter 5 The *Real Poisoning of America – Glycation.*

The Perfect Sugar Ruse

This disturbs me and it disturbs me more and more every day. The company that produces the crop seed for the food I'm supposedly going to eat is the same pharmaceutical company that makes drugs for the illnesses and diseases this food is responsible for? Can this be legal? There's nothing illegal about it, it just happens and you buy into it.

This industry is so intent on keeping us addicted that sugar or corn syrup is quite often the #1 or #2 ingredient in baby food, meaning that if you're not one of the few that were raised on their mother's milk and had to grow up on baby food, you're condemned to an addiction that our grain and pharmaceutical industry has imposed upon you.

It's not surprising that we've ignored this addiction for as long as we've had it. We've ignored it because we grew up with it. Everyone has it, so as far as everyone is concerned, there is no addiction. After all, how can you be addicted to something that you need to survive? How can you live without something that you need to survive? That's where the question lies. Do you need it or not? If it's something you need to survive, why does it do so much damage? Do you really need this food or can you live without it? Allow me to be the first to tell you, you can live without it and you should live without it. To do this, you make your body not need it. Sounds simple, doesn't it? It is simple, it just isn't easy. This is one case where simply is not easy.

We've made it so easy for this industry to increase our addiction that we look forward to finding new ways to inflict more harm on our bodies. And this industry is more than happy to oblige us with their new creations to further our addiction. It's a win-win situation for them. They couldn't ask for anything more. Unfortunately for us, it's a no-win situation. We're paying the supply side for what we eat and the product side for drugs we take to treat what pain the food gives us. This is how Monsanto has engineered the state of your health for their pocketbook.

Monsanto's involvement

According to Wikipedia; *"Monsanto scientists were among the first to genetically modify a plant cell, publishing their results in 1983; five years later, the company conducted the first field tests of genetically engineered crops. Increasing involvement in agricultural biotechnology R&D in general dates from the installment of Richard Mahoney as Monsanto's CEO in 1983 This involvement increased under the leadership of Robert Shapiro, appointed CEO in 1995, leading ultimately to the divestment of product lines unrelated to agriculture."* This divestment of product lines is their disposal of their pharmaceuticals. Their venture into pharmaceuticals started in 1985 with their purchase of GD Searle, of NutraSweet fame. It was eight years after this that they filed for a patent for Celebrex. Did they know at this time, what their food was doing to their consumers? Had they seen any of the reports that started coming out in 1984 and continued until today? Are they aware of any of them now? It appears not, or they're choosing to be electively ignorant. I think it's the latter. Their history tells us it's the latter.

From Wikipedia; *"In 1985, Monsanto acquired G. D. Searle & Company, a life sciences company focusing on pharmaceuticals, agriculture, and animal health. In 1993, Monsanto's Searle division filed a patent application for Celebrex, which in 1998 became the first selective COX-2 inhibitor to be approved by the U.S. Food and Drug Administration (FDA). Celebrex became a blockbuster drug and was often mentioned as a key reason for Pfizer's acquisition of Monsanto's pharmaceutical business in 2002."* Celebrex and arthritis, did they know the connection? What causes arthritis? Was this industry aware of the studies that started coming out in the 50's and 60's about the dangers of their product?

*"In 1996, Monsanto purchased Agracetus, the biotechnology company that had generated the first transgenic varieties of cotton, soybeans, peanuts, and other crops, and from which Monsanto had already been licensing technology since 1991. Monsanto first entered the maize seed business when it purchased 40% of DEKALB in 1996; it purchased the remainder of the corporation in 1998. In 1998 Monsanto purchased Cargill's international seed business, which gave it access to sales and distribution facilities in 51 countries. In 2005, it finalized the purchase of Seminis Inc, a leading global vegetable and fruit seed company, for $1.4 billion. "*This made it the world's largest conventional seed company at the time. Again, I have to wonder, had they seen the studies of what their products were doing to their consumers?

"1999: Monsanto sold off NutraSweet Co. In December, Monsanto merged with Pharmacia and Upjohn. The agricultural division became a wholly owned subsidiary of the "new" Pharmacia; Monsanto's medical research division, which included products such as Celebrex.

"In 2007, Monsanto and BASF announced a long-term agreement to cooperate in the research, development, and marketing of new plant

biotechnology products. "Through a series of transactions, the Monsanto that existed from 1901 to 2000 and the current Monsanto are legally two distinct corporations. Although they share the same name and corporate headquarters, many of the same executives and other employees, and responsibility for liabilities arising out of activities in the industrial chemical business, the agricultural chemicals business is the only segment carried forward from the pre-1997 Monsanto Company to the current Monsanto Company". This was accomplished beginning in the 1980s:

- *1985: Monsanto purchased G. D. Searle & Company for $2.7 billion in cash. In this merger, Searle's aspartame business became a separate Monsanto subsidiary, the NutraSweet Company. CEO of NutraSweet, Robert B. Shapiro, served as CEO of Monsanto from 1995 to 2001.*
- *1996: Monsanto acquired Agracetus, a majority interest in Calgene, creators of the Flavr Savr tomato, and 40% of DeKalb Genetics Corporation. It purchased the remainder of DeKalb in 1998.*
- *1997: Monsanto spun off its industrial chemical and fiber divisions into Solutia. In January, Monsanto announced the purchase of Holden's Foundations Seeds, a privately held seed business. By acquiring Holden's, Monsanto became the biggest American producer of foundation corn, the parent seed from which hybrids are made. The combined purchase price was $925 million. Also, in April, Monsanto purchased the remaining shares of Calgene.*
- *1999: Monsanto sold off NutraSweet Co. In December, Monsanto merged with Pharmacia & Upjohn, and the agricultural division became a wholly owned subsidiary of the "new" Pharmacia; the medical research divisions of Monsanto, which included products such as Celebrex, were rolled into Pharmacia.*
- *2000 (October): Pharmacia spun off its Monsanto subsidiary into a new company, the "new Monsanto". Monsanto agreed to indemnify Pharmacia against any liabilities that might be incurred from judgments against Solutia. As a result, the new Monsanto continues to be a party to numerous lawsuits that relate to operations of the old Monsanto. Pharmacia was bought by Pfizer in a deal announced in 2002 and completed in 2003.)*
- *2005: Monsanto acquired Emergent Genetics and its Stoneville and NexGen cotton brands. Emergent was the third largest U.S. cotton seed company, with about 12 percent of the U.S. market. Monsanto's goal was to obtain "a strategic cotton germplasm and traits platform." The vegetable seed producer Seminis was purchased for $1.4 billion.*
- *2007: In June, Monsanto purchased Delta & Pine Land Company, a major cotton seed breeder, for $1.5 billion. As a condition for approval from the Department of Justice, Monsanto was obligated to divest its Stoneville cotton business, which it sold to Bayer, and to divest its NexGen cotton business, which it sold to Americot. Monsanto also exited the pig breeding business by selling Monsanto Choice Genetics to Newsham Genetics LC*

in November, divesting itself of "any and all swine-related patents, patent applications, and all other intellectual property".

- *2008: Monsanto purchased the Dutch seed company De Ruiter Seeds for €546 million, and sold its POSILAC bovine somatotropin brand and related business to Elanco Animal Health, a division of Eli Lilly in August for $300 million plus "additional contingent consideration".*
- *2012: Monsanto purchased for $210 million Precision Planting Inc., a company that produced computer hardware and software designed to enable farmers to increase yield and productivity through more accurate planting.*
- *2013: Monsanto purchased San Francisco-based Climate Corp for $930 million. Climate Corp. makes more accurate local weather forecasts for farmers based on data modeling and historical data; if the forecasts were wrong, the farmer was recompensed.*
- *2015 Monsanto tried to buy Syngenta for US$46.5 billion but failed.*
- *2016 Bayer offered to buy Monsanto for US$62 billion."*

Monsanto's involvement in the pharmaceutical industry and the AgroSciences has grown to monopolistic proportions. It not only controls what's grown to put on your table to eat, it's made that food so dangerous without you knowing, that it's forcing you to buy their drugs to treat your pain. This forces you into a cycle of their control. It started with the baby food you were given when you were young. It ends with the Ziploc bag full of drugs that your spouse will through away after your death.

It's not just crop seed that they manufacture; they also are responsible for the chemicals sprayed on the crops grown from their seed. Since it's been genetically modified to withstand the effects of their herbicide, Roundup, I've always wondered how much of those chemicals get into our food through this process. Roundup is a glyphosate herbicide, meaning that it's an enzyme inhibitor, that's not good for human health. For me, it's just not healthy enough for me to eat, especially for the problems I already live with. More chemicals in my body are not what I need to keep it healthy. You may want to chance it, but pesticides and herbicides in our diet have been linked to bladder cancer. Why would I want to chance that, just for the taste of something sweet or salty? You only think you're craving the salt when in all actuality, you're craving the carbs that come with the salt. The salt isn't addictive, the carbs are.

Pictured is just a little of Monsanto's bio-chemical industry. They're so good at manufacturing the chemicals for the herbicides and pesticides they manufacture GMO seed that is resistant to these chemicals. This may be good for the crops, but what about you? Though the plant may be resistant to the chemicals, does that mean that your body is? I don't think so.

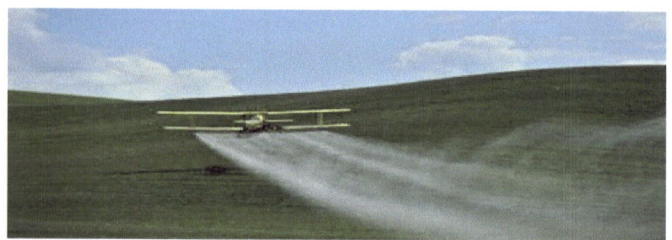

How glyphosate-based herbicides & GM seed combine to make consumption of grains dangerous.

Again according to Wikipedia; *"Monsanto chemist John E. Franz repurposed the chemical glyphosate as a systemic herbicide in 1970. Monsanto's last commercially relevant United States patent on glyphosate expired in 2000, and since then glyphosate has been marketed in the United States and worldwide by many agrochemical companies, in different solution strengths, and with various adjuvants, under dozens of trade names. As of 2009, sales of glyphosate represented about 10% of Monsanto's revenue due to competition from other producers of other glyphosate-based herbicides; their Roundup products (which include GM seeds) represented about half of Monsanto's gross margin."*

Glyphosate is an enzyme inhibitor, used not only in herbicides but also in many drugs. They allow the drug to be more specific to the treatment and incur fewer side effects, for the patient. Don't think that ingestion of Glyphosate now, through your grain intake, will prevent side effects of medications in the future. I can virtually guarantee that it won't.

What Wikipedia says about glyphosate; *"Glyphosate is absorbed through foliage, and minimally through roots, and transported to growing points. It inhibits a plant enzyme involved in the synthesis of three aromatic amino acids: tyrosine, tryptophan, and phenylalanine. Therefore, it is effective only on actively growing plants and is not effective as a pre-emergence herbicide. An increasing number of crops have been genetically engineered to be tolerant of glyphosate (e.g. Roundup Ready soybean, the first Roundup Ready crop, also created by Monsanto) which allows farmers to use glyphosate as a post-emergence herbicide against weeds. The development of glyphosate resistance in weed species is emerging as a costly problem. While glyphosate and formulations such as Roundup have been approved by regulatory bodies worldwide, concerns about their effects on humans and the environment persist."*

"Many regulatory and scholarly reviews have evaluated the relative toxicity of glyphosate as an herbicide. The German Federal Institute for Risk Assessment toxicology review in 2013 found that "the available data is

contradictory and far from being convincing" with regard to correlations between exposure to glyphosate formulations and risk of various cancers, including non-Hodgkin lymphoma *(NHL)."*

A 2014 review article reported a significant association between B-cell lymphoma and glyphosate occupational exposure. In March 2015 the World Health Organization's International Agency for Research on Cancer classified glyphosate as *"probably carcinogenic in humans" (category 2A) based on epidemiological studies, animal studies, and in vitro studies. However in 2016 a joint meeting of the United Nations (FAO) Panel of Experts on Pesticide Residues in Food and the Environment and the World Health Organization (WHO) Core Assessment Group on Pesticide Residues (JMPR) concluded that based on the available evidence "glyphosate is unlikely to pose a carcinogenic risk to humans from exposure through the diet".* This last statement I wonder about. It also makes me wonder, "who influenced their decision to label this stuff as suitable to eat?" Apparently, they're not taking the rise in cancer rates into consideration.

Are you glyphosate-resistant? Can your body withstand the changes that glyphosate forces upon your body every time you have a corn chip or a sandwich? With Roundup being coated on most of the foods that you eat, how can you guarantee that none of it is in your body? How can you guarantee that it's not affecting your physiology? Can you guarantee that it's not affecting the actions of enzymes in your body that regulate your health? What guarantees do you have that this won't initiate more trips to your doctor?

What you think may not be of much importance, maybe far more important that you believe. Acetylcholine is an important chemical in the body that's important for brain function and muscle function throughout the body as Acetylcholine is a neurotransmitter. For Acetylcholine to act as a neurotransmitter, it needs multiple enzymes that function in the central nervous system and the peripheral nervous system. Acetylcholine works as a neurotransmitter as well as a neuromodulator.

The body uses the enzyme acetylcholinesterase to help activate muscles by inhibiting the action of acetylcholine, and if glyphosate herbicides (Roundup weed killer) are enzyme inhibitors, how can the ingestion of grains laden with these herbicides, not affect the function of the enzymes in your body since you consume them every time you eat bread products of any sort? Corn chips and soy fall into this category also. (They may be worse.)

These Glyphosate herbicides are enzyme inhibitors that have the ability to alter or stop the cell signaling capabilities of enzymes. If they can do this to plants, where is the guarantee that it won't affect your body? Chances are, they're going to change how your body operates and in the long run be the precursor to many diseases. It's crucial for the body's proper function that the actions of certain enzymes are never altered. Where's the guarantee that these enzyme-inhibiting herbicides that your wheat has been sprayed with, won't affect your health? There is none except that if you eat this food, you will be affected.

According to Wikipedia; *"Acetylcholine receptor agonists and antagonists can either have an effect directly on the receptors or exert their effects indirectly, e.g., by affecting the enzyme acetylcholinesterase, which degrades the receptor ligand. Agonists increase the level of receptor activation, antagonists reduce it."* I would consider an enzyme inhibitor an antagonist as it inhibits enzyme function.

It's a little clearer to see now, how the altering of how enzymes work in our bodies, can have an effect on our health. I can see how this could come from a diet high in grains because of how much Roundup is sprayed on grain that's milled into flour. I can also see how this could present a huge gain for the pharmaceutical industry. Is this really the intent of Monsanto, the maker of Roundup, the widest used herbicide on the planet? Or is it just negligence? I have to wonder because of their previous ties with Pharmacia & Upjohn, makers of Celebrex. These are just a few of thousands of enzymes and cell signaling proteins that are affected by this enzyme inhibitor. How many corporate breakups don't include severance packages that include stock options? Is this what makes Monsanto want to continue their glyphosate spraying?

I for one, would not like to have this inhibitor flowing through my blood mucking up my system. Who knows what enzymes it's going to inhibit in your body? Fortunately for me, I don't have to worry about that anymore, as carbs aren't in my diet. They won't get a chance to muck up anything in my body ever again, I've gone keto and I'm not going back.

It looks to me like Monsanto is trying to lock up not only our digestive problems but the resolve of those digestive problems as well. They like to persuade you to buy their food products which you are more than happy to do, then they get your money again when you purchase your Celebrex to ease the pain of arthritis given you by their grains. The next step is to buy their drugs to counteract the side effects of the original drug you need to take for the pain. You don't want to know the step after that, my dad can tell you, it's not pretty and it involves, even more, drugs and more therapy and continued testing. It's a never-ending cycle that lasts until death.

Bayer's involvement

"It's not only Monsanto, Bayer has its own interest in the area of crop science, as explained by Wikipedia, " in 2002, Bayer AG acquired the Dutch

seed company Nunhems, which at the time was one of the world's top five seed companies. In 2006, the U.S. Department of Agriculture announced that Bayer CropScience's Liberty Link genetically modified rice had contaminated the U.S. rice supply. Shortly after the public learned of the contamination, the E.U. banned imports of U.S. long-grain rice and the futures price plunged. In April 2010, a Lonoke County, Arkansas jury awarded a dozen farmers $48 million. The case is currently on appeal to the Arkansas Supreme Court. On 1 July 2011 Bayer CropScience agreed to a global settlement for up to $750 million. In September 2014, the firm announced plans to invest $1 billion in the United States between 2013 and 2016. A Bayer spokesperson said that the largest investments will be made to expand the production of its herbicide Liberty. Liberty is used to kill weeds which have grown resistant to Monsanto's product Roundup."

Bayer's four divisions are related in their concerns to their contribution to our food industry as well as their contribution to the pharmaceutical industry. Bayer Pharmaceuticals, Bayer Crop Science, Bayer Animal Health, and Bayer Consumer Health are all related to our health. They too, like to charge us for the food they market to us, then charge us for medication to treat the symptoms of the diseases that their foods are responsible for. Their divested interests are Lanxess (Bayer Chemicals AG) Diagnostics Division, Diabetes Devices Division, Covestro (Bayer Material Science).

Astra Zenica / Syngenta's involvement

"Zeneca Agrochemicals was part of AstraZeneca, and formerly of Imperial Chemical Industries. ICI was formed in the UK in 1926. Two years later, work began at the Agricultural Research Station at Jealotts Hill near Bracknell." "In 2004, Syngenta Seeds purchased Garst, the North American corn and soybean business of Advanta, as well as Golden Harvest Seeds. On 5 December 2004, the European Union ended a six-year moratorium when it approved imports of two varieties of genetically modified corn sold by Monsanto and its Swiss rival, Syngenta.

AstraZeneca owned by Syngenta again is evidence of this industrial control over our lives. Syngenta is a Swiss biotechnology company that operates globally. According to Wikipedia; "Syngenta AG is a global Swiss agribusiness that produces agrochemicals and seeds. As a biotechnology company, it conducts genomic research. It was formed in 2000 by the merger of Novartis Agribusiness and Zeneca Agrochemicals. As of 2014, Syngenta was the world's largest crop chemical producer, strongest in Europe. As of 2009, it ranked third in seeds and biotechnology sales. Sales in 2015 were approximately US$13.4 billion, over half of which were in emerging markets."

The three agrichemical companies above are the largest in the world, controlling a majority of the foods we eat along with the medications we take. I've laid out the evidence of what their foods do to the human body, yet they continue to produce the seed for the crops to make the food they want us to put on our table to eat. They also produce the aspirin everybody takes for the headaches they get from eating their bread.

I've said before how convenient we've made it for this industry to take our money while slowly, painfully, and expensively, make us sick. But our money is not the only thing they rob us of. They rob us of our dignity as well, for their food does more than anything else to rob us of our memories. We allow them to do this because none of their foods require warning labels, like that of cigarettes. (The FDA doesn't seem to care about what it does to you, they only care that you know it's there, even though you don't know what it's doing to you.) Even the USDA's *myplate.gov* still recommends eating them.

We've put our health and lives in the hands of this industry by bending to their advertising and buying into their game. We allow them to addict us when we're infants by dumping sugar and corn syrup solids into the baby food we feed our kids. Then we allow them to continue their assault by buying into advertising schemes every Saturday morning with their cereal commercials. To fully hook us, they add sugar to this already sugar-laden food simply to make it more palatable.

When an industry does this, how are we supposed to fight the addiction? This makes every American who buys into this behavior a slave to this industry. Slaves make the best captive audience. They have no choice in what they do except to choose their device of demise. Will it be corn flakes or Wheaties?

What more do you need than a captive audience to sell your wares? This is why a Coke at a ballgame costs 3 times more than what you can get it for, at the grocery store. At the ballgame, you're a captive audience. It's the same when you're addicted. Every 'PUSHER' knows this and they charge a premium price for it. This is exactly why everyone who remains in this trap makes themselves a slave, captive to the whims of these industries.

The Litigation Game

These industries are tied up with multiple lawsuits in other areas of their agrochemical businesses. For example, Monsanto has fought legal claims of false advertising, as explained again in Wikipedia;

1. "In 1999, Monsanto was condemned by the UK Advertising
    Standards Authority (ASA) for making "confusing, misleading,
    unproven and wrong" claims about its products over the course of a
    £1 million advertising campaign. The ASA ruled that Monsanto had
    presented its opinions "as accepted fact" and had published "wrong"
    and "unproven" scientific claims. Monsanto responded with an
    apology and claimed it was not intending to deceive and instead "did

not take sufficiently into account the difference in culture between the UK and the USA in the way some of this information was presented."

2. *"In 2001, French environmental and consumer rights campaigners brought a case against Monsanto for misleading the public about the environmental impact of its herbicide Roundup, on the basis that glyphosate, Roundup's main ingredient, is classed as "dangerous for the environment" and "toxic for aquatic organisms" by the European Union. Monsanto's advertising for Roundup had presented it as biodegradable and as leaving the soil clean after use. In 2007, Monsanto was convicted of false advertising and was fined 15,000 Euros. Monsanto's French distributor Scotts France was also fined 15,000 Euros. Both defendants were ordered to pay damages of 5,000 Euros to the Brittany Water and Rivers Association and 3,000 Euros to the CLCV (Consommation Logement Cadre de vie), one of the two main general consumer associations in France. Monsanto appealed and the court upheld the verdict; Monsanto appealed again to the French Supreme Court, and in 2009 it also upheld the verdict.*

3. *"In August 2012, a Brazilian Regional Federal Court ordered Monsanto to pay a $250,000 fine for false advertising. In 2004, advertising that related to the use of GM soya seed, and the herbicide glyphosate used in its cultivation, claimed it was beneficial to the conservation of the environment. The federal prosecutor maintained that Monsanto misrepresented the amount of herbicide required and stated that "there is no scientific certainty that soybeans marketed by Monsanto use less herbicide." The presiding judge condemned Monsanto and called the advertisement "abusive and misleading propaganda." The prosecutor held that the goal of the advertising was to prepare the market for the purchase of genetically modified soybean seed (sale of which was then banned) and the herbicide used on it, at a time when the approval of a Brazilian Biosafety Law, enacted in 2005, was being discussed in the country."*

4. *"In March 2014 the South African Advertising Standards Authority (ASA) upheld a complaint, made by the African Centre for Biosafety, that Monsanto had made "unsubstantiated" claims about genetically modified crops in its radio advertisements, and ordered that these adverts be pulled. In March 2015 after considering further documentation from Monsanto, the ASA reversed its ruling."*

5. *"In 2009, Monsanto came under scrutiny from the U.S. Department of Justice, which began investigating whether the company's activities in the soybean markets were breaking anti-trust rules. In*

2010, the Department of Justice created a website through which comments on "Agriculture and Antitrust Enforcement Issues in Our 21st Century Economy" could be submitted; over 15,000 comments were submitted including a letter by 14 State Attorneys General. The comments are publicly available. On November 16, 2012, Monsanto announced that it had received written notification from the U.S. Department of Justice that the Antitrust Division had concluded its inquiry and that the Department of Justice had closed the inquiry without taking any enforcement action. Opponents of Monsanto's seed patenting and licensing practices expressed frustration that the Department of Justice released no information about the results of the inquiry.

6.   *"In 2009, Monsanto came under scrutiny from the U.S. Department of Justice, which began investigating whether the company's activities in the soybean markets were breaking anti-trust rules. In 2010, the Department of Justice created a website through which comments on "Agriculture and Antitrust Enforcement Issues in Our 21st Century Economy" could be submitted; over 15,000 comments were submitted including a letter by 14 State Attorneys General. The comments are publicly available. On November 16, 2012, Monsanto announced that it had received written notification from the U.S. Department of Justice that the Antitrust Division had concluded its inquiry and that the Department of Justice had closed the inquiry without taking any enforcement action. Opponents of Monsanto's seed patenting and licensing practices expressed frustration that the Department of Justice released no information about the results of the inquiry."*

This is a normal operating business for Monsanto, Syngenta, and Bayer. Too bad it isn't for you. All of these cases are a clear indication of the extent to which Monsanto is willing to push the limits. This is how corporate risk/loss assessment works. Sometimes the risk of paying a $15,000 find is worth the theft of a patent. My problem with this is they playing with my health. If I decide to eat their products, I get to play their game of disease and drugs. The problem is, what are their products? Who knows? Who knows who grow the crops for the corn flakes that you ate this morning for breakfast. Do you? I don't. But I now know it came from one of these companies.

Monsanto's not the only one. Syngenta, as well, has been accused of making false claims about being involved in suits for false patent infringement;

"In 2001, the United States Patent and Trademark Office ruled in favor of Syngenta which had filed a suit against Bayer for patent infringement on a class of neonicotinoid insecticides. The following year Syngenta filed suits against Monsanto and other companies claiming infringement of its U.S.

biotechnology patents covering genetically modified corn and cotton. In 2004, it again filed a suit against Monsanto, claiming antitrust violations related to the U.S. biotech corn seed market, and Monsanto countersued. Monsanto and Syngenta settled all litigation in 2008"

I mention this to point out the extent of their influence in the crop seed industry, where they have 15 of their own seed companies that all provide GMO crop seed for farmers to plant for their crops for food which ends up on our tables. Syngenta is the second largest corporation in the industry, Monsanto is even larger. (And we haven't considered Bayer CropScience, Dow AgroSciences or DuPont Pioneer.) Most of these cases involve patent rights to GMO seed with companies like Monsanto or DuPont Pioneer. It's not just patent problems that their litigation deals with; most of these companies like to make out that their chemical products are completely harmless to the environment when they've been proven otherwise.

"Syngenta was a defendant in a class action lawsuit by the city of Greenville, Illinois concerning the adverse effects of atrazine in human water supplies. The suit was settled for $105 million in May 2012. A similar case involving six states has been in federal court since 2010." "In the US, Syngenta is facing lawsuits from farmers and shipping companies regarding Viptera genetically modified corn. The plaintiffs in nearly 30 states contend that Syngenta's introduction of Viptera drove down US grain market prices, leading to financial harm and that Syngenta acted irresponsibly by doing too little to enable shipping companies to export the grain to approved ports. Before Vipera's 2010 introduction Syngenta secured all US and NCGA-recommended export approvals, but none from China. China had imported little to no US grain prior to 2010, and at the time was not considered a major partner, but it became a major partner in 2010 when it dramatically increased US grain imports. For three years, China imported U.S. Viptera grain without formal approval. In November 2013, Chinese officials destroyed a U.S. grain shipment containing Viptera grain, started rejecting all US shipments with the GM grain, but continued to accept it from all countries other than the US. That same year, US corn market prices dropped $4 per bushel, causing over $2.9B in losses, with just over half of that loss occurring prior to China's November rejection. China later approved the GM corn in 2014 but US corn grain market prices have not rebounded."

I can only empathize with the farmers and the losses they've had to sustain. Their losses, fortunately, were only monetary. How many others have suffered losses of family members, like my family? Our losses were not only financial, they were family. It would be nice if money or the bottom line wasn't the most important thing in the industry. But it is. And we have to live with it. My choice is to not buy into it. I won't eat what they grow or take their drugs to fix the problems caused by what they grow. My choice is a choice of survival.

These are the kind of companies that are ultimately providing your food. Do you want them making your drugs, also? As you've seen, they already do. Do you wonder why the prevalence of these diseases is so rampant? It's in these industries' best interest that this cycle continues. Do you want this kind of industry to be responsible for your food or medicine? How about the medicine they make to treat the problems their foods create? We've allowed this to take place, right under our noses and we should be ashamed. Doesn't this sound a lot like a wicked witch luring small children with candy and sweets? Because of our addiction, we allow them to continue this behavior.

This addiction has and is costing America more money and lives than any other addiction that we've ever experienced. There are 24,000,000 deaths worldwide each year due to ECC, excessive carbohydrate consumption. There were 17.3 million deaths in 2013 alone due to cardiovascular disease. Cancer claims over 4 million each year and Alzheimer's take 5 million each year, yet I hear no outrage about it. All of these deaths and suffering can be curbed simply by curbing carbohydrate consumption.

It's time to put an end to this addiction. It's time for a cure. But to stop the addiction, you first have to de-celebratize it. We have to stop celebrating its addictive qualities and exchange that celebration for the horror for what this addiction really does.

Everybody needs to think about what harm this food does before they put it in their mouth instead of thinking how good it tastes. Unfortunately for my generation and all those that have come along since, we're stuck in the quagmire of addiction that we have to carry for the rest of our lives. Even most natural causes of death happen in part, due to what this food has done to the body over the lifetime of the deceased. An autopsy will likely show some form of arthritis, as this is evidence of inflammation, oxidative stress and cell degradation that these foods cause. If the inflammation, oxidative stress and cell degradation exists in the joints, it has to exist elsewhere in the body and since it exists throughout the body, as inflammation exists in the blood, it has to affect everything it comes in contact with.

That means it affects your heart, your brain, and every internal organ. How can that not have an effect on your life? It has to, so I have to ask, why is this food still allowed to be sold without a warning about just how dangerous it is? Cigarettes are and require a warning. Alcohol is and it requires a warning also. Heroin is illegal and opioids require prescriptions. But not the one substance that minimizes all the damage caused by these other substances collectively, sugar from grains requires any warning for the damage it inflicts. Why is this not as important? Is this industry too big to fail? Is there a way they can change it? I for one, cannot wait, I can't afford to play their game.

Going back to the problems this industry has had in court, mostly protecting their own patents and falsely claiming that their products are nutritious when they're not. Most of the patent problems lie in the resistance their new crop seeds have to their pesticides and herbicides, which have proven to have adverse effects on the human body. Yet they are still allowed to spray their crops with these herbicides and pesticides. My question is, how much of these herbicides and pesticides trickle into our food supply? How confident are you that no chemicals are in what you eat? How confident are you that no enzyme controlling chemicals are not on your biscuits or crackers? How confident are you that your sugar addiction won't turn into diabetes? How confident are you that your addiction won't turn into heart disease or cancer? Whether you worry about it or not, you will experience brain loss. That's just in the science. You can't change it without saying goodbye to your addiction. This obviously isn't easy with a grain industry that feeds the pharmaceutical industry. It's even more obvious that they'll never let us know the damage their foods do to everyone who ingests them. That's up to you to know the dangers of sugar and grains, and now you do.

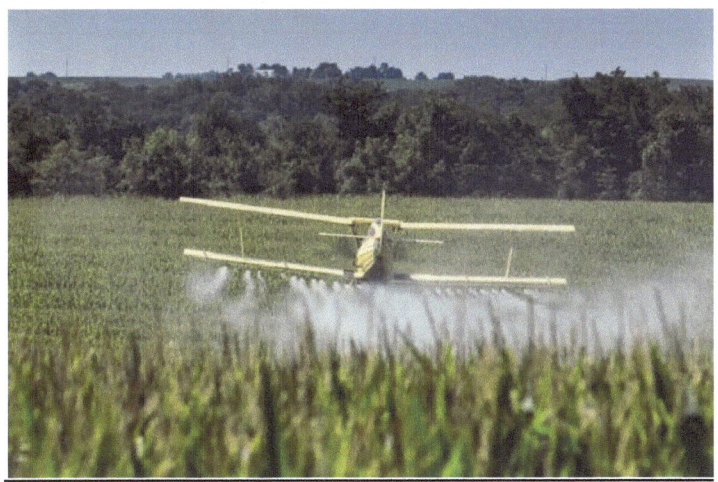

Do You Know Everything About What You're Eating?

Would you eat it if you did?

PART II

THE INESCAPABLE DAMAGE

THE DESTINY OF GRAINS IN THE DIET

Your Carb Diet Brings This Destruction,

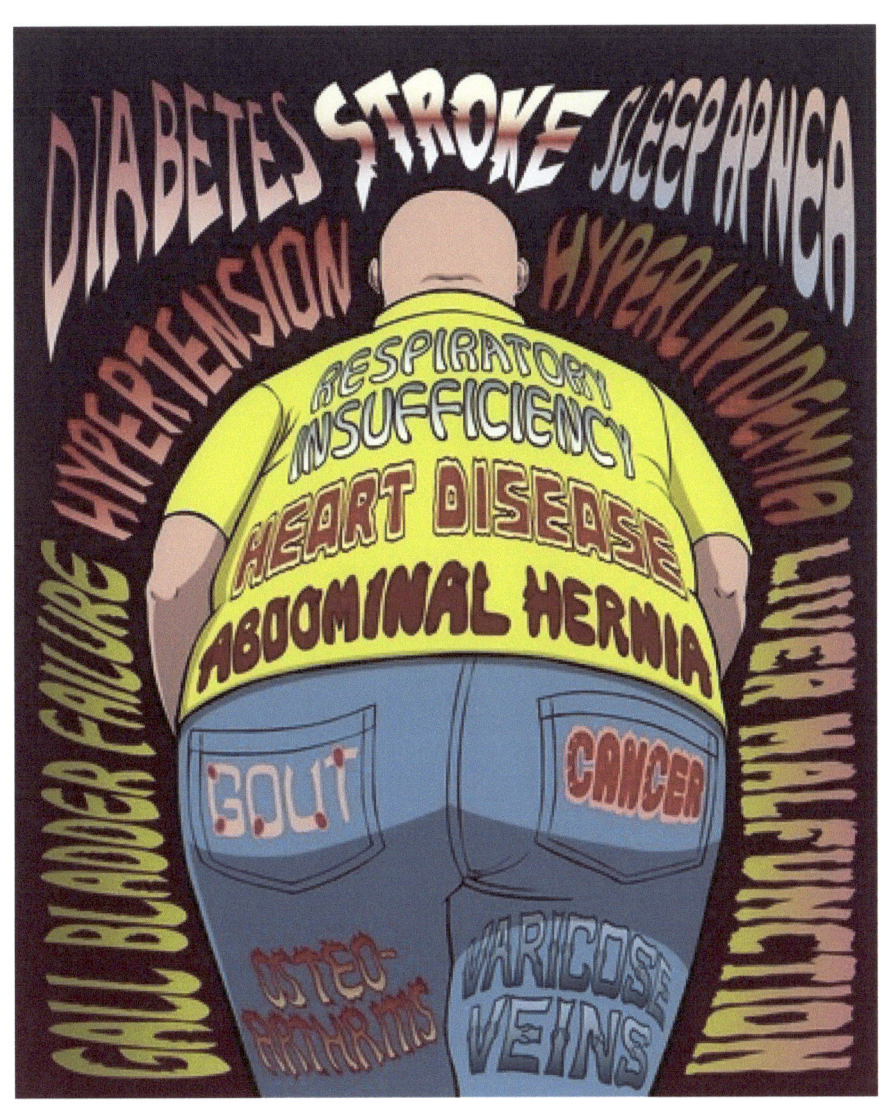

Unless You Change the Pattern,

Your Poison Will Pick You

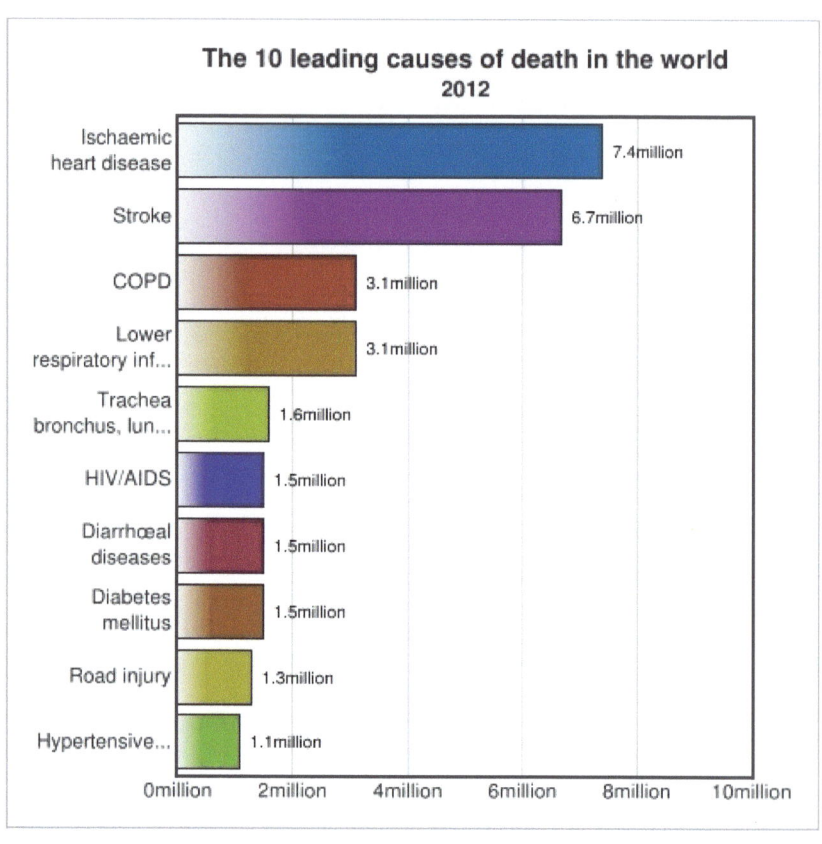

The 10 leading causes of death in the world
2012

Ischaemic heart disease	7.4 million
Stroke	6.7 million
COPD	3.1 million
Lower respiratory inf...	3.1 million
Trachea bronchus, lun...	1.6 million
HIV/AIDS	1.5 million
Diarrhœal diseases	1.5 million
Diabetes mellitus	1.5 million
Road injury	1.3 million
Hypertensive...	1.1 million

7 of the above 10 causes of death are a direct result of ECC, Excessive Carbohydrate Consumption, something you have the power to change

CHAPTER 4

Diseases Caused By the Formation of Plaque in Your Body

Plaque is arguably the worst manifestation of glycation from sugar and carbs in the diet. It happens when a sugar molecule combines with any fat or protein molecule, (including hemoglobin) without a cell signaling protein (hormone) to tell it what to do. It besets the true destructive force of glucose on your body. This is why insulin is so important. It's that cell signaling protein, a hormone, in this case, that tells glucose to turn into fat, so it can be used as fuel. Without the insulin, the glucose is free to attach its polymer base molecule to any protein or lipid (usually an LDL particle or hemoglobin protein in your blood), to start the process of glycation.

Whether the glycation is of a lipid or a protein, which is always the case when it comes in contact with cholesterol, especially LDL particles, the resulting glycation usually ends up in the form of a plaque, macrophages, and cytokines. There are several forms of plaque. According to Wikipedia, there are seven different kinds of plaque, Amyloid Plaque, Atheroma Plaque, Dental plaque, Mucoid plaque, Pleural plaque, Senile plaques, Viral plaque.

By far the worst of the plaques caused by digesting wheat and gluten is amyloid plaque, because of all the diseases it has a role in. According to Wikipedia;

"Amyloids are insoluble fibrous protein aggregates *sharing specific structural traits. They are insoluble and arise from at least 18 inappropriately folded versions of proteins and* polypeptides *present naturally in the body. These misfolded structures alter their proper configuration such that they erroneously interact with one another or other cell components forming insoluble* fibrils. *They have been associated with the pathology of more than 20 serious human diseases in that abnormal accumulation of amyloid fibrils in organs may lead to* amyloidosis, *and may play a role in various neurodegenerative disorders. "The list of diseases caused by amyloid plaque is quite extensive, ranging from Alzheimer's disease to Diabetes, Parkinson's and Huntington's diseases and more.*

The list on Wikipedia is 21 diseases and disorders or conditions associated with amyloid plaque. In my opinion, amyloid plaque is caused by the digestion of gluten from any source, whether it's wheat, barley or rye.

Wikipedia says;
"Studies have shown that amyloid deposition is associated with mitochondrial dysfunction and a resulting generation of reactive oxygen species *(ROS), which can initiate a signaling pathway leading to* apoptosis.*"*

In short amyloid plaque is caused by oxidative stress and cell death, both of which are caused by consumption of gluten and other high starch products.

Atheromatous Plaques *are basically plaques from fats and is the type of plaque that clogs up your artery walls. This is the type of plaque that causes* atherosclerosis *and leads to heart and cardiovascular disease. It is the root cause of high blood pressure.*
Dental plaque is caused by the excessive amount of sugar on the teeth, creating bacteria, causing decay.

Remember, carbs = sugar, and saliva is a major enzyme for digestion called α-amylase, an important enzyme for breaking down starches. This is the enzyme that starts glycation. If plaque from glycation can accumulate on your teeth, this is a sign of glycation starting even before you can swallow.

"Senile plaques (also known as neuritic plaques, senile druse and brain druse) are extracellular deposits of amyloid beta in the grey matter of the brain. They're responsible for diseases such as Alzheimer's disease and dementia, and play a role in most every other cognitive disorder due to the way this plaque gums up the neurons in your brain.
"Mucoid plaque (or mucoid cap or rope) is a pseudoscientific term used by some alternative medicine *advocates to describe what is claimed to be a combination of allegedly harmful mucus-like material and food residue that they say coats the* gastrointestinal tract *of most people. The term was coined by Richard Anderson, a naturopath, and entrepreneur, who sells a range of products that claim to "cleanse" the body of such purported plaques."*
Pleural plaques are indicators of asbestos *exposure and the most common asbestos-induced lesion. They usually appear after 20 years or more of exposure and degenerate into* mesothelioma. *They appear as fibrous plaques on the parietal* pleura, *usually on both sides, and at the posterior and inferior part of the chest wall as well as the diaphragm.*

With atherosclerosis being arguably the worst of these manifestations as it's at the root of most heart disease and cardiovascular disease, the plaque that creates this atherosclerosis earns itself #1 in the death and destruction category. Since this comes mostly from sugar and grains, both products of Monsanto's farmers, you can thank Monsanto for your cancers and CVDs, your arthritis and IBS, your diabetes and your pancreatitis. The list can keep going on and on and on. It's the gluten that breaks down into glucose to create that glycation. This was shown in a 1984 study, yet the practice continued and even escalated to the point of where it is today. With all this plaque caused by glycation, I have to wonder why this food hasn't been condemned yet.

According to Wikipedia; *"The formation and accumulation of advanced glycation endproducts (AGEs) have been implicated in the progression of age-related diseases. AGEs have been implicated in Alzheimer's disease, cardiovascular disease, and stroke. The mechanism by which AGEs induce damage is through a process called cross-linking that causes intracellular damage and apoptosis. They form photosensitizers in the crystalline lens, which has implications for cataract development. Reduced muscle function is also associated with AGEs."*

What it boils down to is this;

Sugar causes glycation. Glycation causes inflammation. Inflammation is responsible for most pain in your body as well as most disease in your body Including:

- diabetes
- Hypertension
- hyperlipidemia
- atherosclerosis
- Inflammatory heart disease
- Inflammatory Bowel syndrome
- Every form of cancer
- Alzheimer's disease
- Parkinson's disease
- Schizophrenia
- Depression
- Bipolar disorder
- arthritis
- Chronic Pain
- Headaches

If you could eliminate all of the above disorders by limiting the amount of cholesterol that's glycated into plaque, wouldn't you consider that at least a step toward a cure? By that logic, wouldn't limiting the amount of glucose you put in your body limit the amount of glycation and plaque in your blood since it's the glucose that does the glycating? This is something that you have full control over how it affects your body.

Failure to Control Your Glucose Intake

Brings You to Your Destiny; Glycation

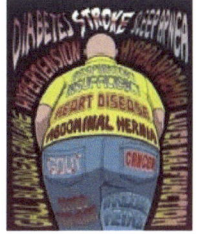

Chapter 5

Glycation - The Real Poisoning of America

Of the causes of death below from Wikipedia, Ischaemic heart disease @ 7.4 million ranks right at the top. This is the result of glycation, 5 of the following 8 are also caused by non-enzymatic glycation. Hence my proposal, control the glycation and you control all modern diseases.

According to Wikipedia;

*Leading causes of preventable death worldwide as of the year 2001, according to researchers working with the Disease Control Priorities Network (DCPN) and the World Health Organization (WHO). (THE WHO'S **2008 statistics** SHOW VERY SIMILAR TRENDS.)* Imagine what they are right now, 8 years later and what they will be eight years from now if nothing is

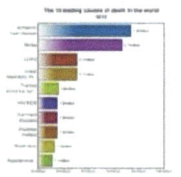 done about it. Think it might be time for a cure?

The top 10 causes of preventable death, ones influenced by glycation are in red. Although it may be difficult to stop all glycation in the body, due to its commonality, you can control a major portion of it. Excessive Carbohydrate Consumption, the primary cause of glycation is controllable. Failure to control your consumption leads directly to any of the following disorders in red ;

1. Ischaemic heart disease @ 7.4 mil
2. Stroke@ 6.7 mil
3. COPD @ 3.1 mil
4. Lower Respiratory infection @ 3.1mil
5. Trachea bronchus, lung infection@1.6 mil
6. HIV/AIDS@1.5 mil
7. Diarrheal diseases@1.5 mil
8. Diabetes mellitus@1.5 mil
9. Road injury@1.3 mil
10. Hypertension@1.1 mil

85% of these deaths or 24.5 million are directly linked to **ECC,** Excessive Carbohydrate Consumption, making them the most preventable causes of death. 24.5 million deaths each and every year amounts to over 67,123 people each and every day. That includes approximately 2684 Americans each and every day. We have full control of this. All it would take is to say no to the sugar and grain industries. This one response would allow over 2680 more Americans to stay alive, every day. The cessation of carb consumption could add an additional 10-20 years to their lives, simply by eliminating the primary cause of inflammation, glucose. The continuation of carb consumption will, by contrast, prove the destructive power of sugar, by eventually killing all of its hosts.

Glycation is a common everyday experience that you accelerate with a carbohydrate diet. The more carbs you eat, the more glycation you'll get to deal with. Glycation is controllable by controlling what you put in your mouth to eat. Although not totally responsible for some of these cancers, they would not exist if the glycation didn't exist. This is the basis of my contention that if you eliminate the reason for the glycation, you eliminate the reason for inflammation, which in turn will eliminate the reason for these diseases, thereby eliminating the disease. It's really not hard to see, once you take a good look at it; carb consumption is responsible for the inflammation that builds in the blood that is responsible for 90% of all modern diseases. Remove the inflammation by removing the sugar, which means removing the carbs. A simpler solution doesn't exist and this cure can be yours.

These Are Some of the Smoking Gun Articles of Evidence

That the FDA and the USDA Are Ignoring.

They Put Your Health and Life at **Risk, By Doing So.**

50 of the 17676 studies done on glycation are below. These research studies were chosen from 281 studies that I examined for evidence of what glycation does to the body. By going through only 2% of these studies, I was able to find enough damning evidence to condemn this food 31 times over. By this ratio, I'll end up finding at the least 1950 more studies showing damage that glycation does.

I chose to search glycation because I know that it's at the root of all modern diseases from cancer to CVDs to arthritis to dementia including Alzheimer disease. The following studies are the proof of what glycation does, and with sugar being the primary instigator of glycation, removal of sugar from the diet will eliminate everything it's responsible for. **These AGEs are responsible for all modern diseases and thus, are the reason for this book.** When you eat carbs, you need to know what those carbs do to your body.

The study that piqued my interest initially was the report on RAGEs, this report dated Jun 5, 2011, can be found in PubMed at *Receptor for advanced glycation end-products- mediated inflammation and diabetic vascular complications.* It explains how glycation turns your body's fuel (cholesterol) and proteins (hemoglobin) into AGEs before they can be used for fuel and body repair.

Receptor for advanced glycation end products

"Exposure of amino residue of proteins to reducing sugars, such as glucose, glucose 6-phosphate, fructose, ribose and intermediate aldehydes, results in non-enzymatic glycation, which forms reversible Schiff bases and Amadori compounds. A series of further complex molecular rearrangements then yield irreversible advanced glycation end-products (AGE). The aldehydes, highly reactive AGE precursors, are produced by both enzymatic and non-enzymatic pathways. The enzymatic pathways include a route of myeloperoxidase in inflammatory cells, such as activated macrophages, which produces hypochlorite, then reacting with serine to generate glycolaldehyde." Study Link

The following report from Oct 27, 2016, is the evidence of glucose's involvement in arthritis. By being responsible for glycation, the glucose from broken down carbs, again, is directly responsible for arthritis, just like it was in the 4,000 yr old ice mummy recovered from a receding glacier.

"Protein oxidation, nitration and glycation biomarkers for early-stage diagnosis of osteoarthritis of the knee and typing and progression of arthritic disease"

"Glycated, oxidized and nitrated proteins and amino acids were detected in synovial fluid and plasma of arthritic patients with characteristic patterns found in early and advanced OA and RA, and non-RA, with respect to healthy controls. In early-stage disease, two algorithms for consecutive use in diagnosis were developed: (1) disease versus healthy control, and (2) classification as OA, RA, and non-RA." Study Link
The following report from Sep 23, 2016, shows the effects that AGEs have on the body in the diseases it promotes.

"Effect of glycation inhibitors on aging and age-related diseases"
"Vast evidence supports the view that glycation of proteins is one of the main factors contributing to aging and is an important element of etiopathology of age-related diseases, especially type 2 diabetes mellitus, cataract, and neurodegenerative diseases. Counteracting glycation can, therefore, be a means of increasing both the lifespan and health span. In this review, accumulation of glycation products during aging is presented, pathophysiological effects of glycation are discussed and ways of attenuation of the effects of glycation are described, concentrating on prevention of glycation. The effects of glycation and glycation inhibitors on the course of selected age-related diseases, such as Alzheimer's disease, Parkinson's disease, and cataract are also reviewed." Study Link
This study from Oct 21, 2016, looks at the damaging effects of glycation along with the protective effects of certain phytochemicals (anti-oxidant producing agents).

"Phytochemicals against advanced glycation end products (AGEs) and the receptor system"

"Reducing sugars can react non-enzymatically with amino groups of proteins and lipids to form irreversibly cross-linked macro protein derivatives called as advanced glycation end products (AGEs). Cross-linking modification of extracellular matrix proteins by AGEs deteriorate their tertiary structural integrity and function, contributing to aging-related organ damage and diabetes-associated complications, such as cardiovascular disease (CVD). Moreover, engagement of receptor for AGEs, RAGE with the ligands evoke oxidative stress generation and inflammatory, thrombotic and fibrotic reactions in various kinds of tissues, further exacerbating the deleterious effects of AGEs on multiple organ systems. So the AGE-RAGE axis is a novel therapeutic target for numerous devastating disorders. Several observational studies have shown the association of dietary consumption of fruits and vegetables with the reduced risk of CVD in a general population. Although beneficial effects of fruits and vegetables against CVD could mainly be ascribed to its anti-oxidative properties, blockade of the AGE-RAGE axis by phytochemicals may also contribute to cardiovascular event protection. Therefore, in this review, we focus on 4 phytochemicals (quercetin, sulforaphane, iridoids, and curcumin) and summarize their effects on AGE formation as well as RAGE-mediated signaling pathway in various cell types and organs, including endothelial cells, vessels, and heart."

This report from Sep 16, 2016, examines the nature of amyloid plaque and glyoxal *(Glyoxal is an inflammatory compound formed when cooking oils and fats are heated to high temperatures).* It's also made in your body when your body breaks down glucose.

"Glyoxal administration induces formation of high molecular weight aggregates of hemoglobin exhibiting amyloidal nature in experimental rats: An in vivo study"

"Glyoxal, a highly reactive α-oxoaldehyde, increases in diabetic condition and reacts with proteins to form advanced glycation end products (AGEs). In the present study, we have investigated the effect of glyoxal on experimental rat hemoglobin in vivo after external administration of the α-dicarbonyl compound in animals. Gel electrophoretic profile of hemolysate collected from glyoxal-treated rats (32mg/kg body wt. dose) after one week exhibited the presence of some high molecular weight protein bands that were found to be absent for control, untreated rats. Mass spectrometric and absorption studies indicated that the bands represented hemoglobin. Further studies revealed that the fraction exhibited the presence of intermolecular cross β-sheet structure. Thus glyoxal administration induces the formation of high molecular weight aggregates of hemoglobin with amyloid characteristics in rats. Aggregated hemoglobin fraction was found to exhibit higher stability compared to glyoxal-untreated hemoglobin. As evident from mass spectrometric studies, glyoxal was found to modify Arg-30β and Arg-31α of rat hemoglobin to hydroimidazolone adducts. The modifications thus appear

to induce amyloid-like aggregation of hemoglobin in rats. Considering the increased level of glyoxal in diabetes mellitus as well as its high reactivity, the above findings may be physiologically significant.

In view of its inflammatory function in innate immunity and its ability to detect a class of ligands through a common structural motif, rage is often referred to as a pattern recognition receptor." Study link

This report from Oct 18, 2016, examines the relationship of high mobility group box 1 (HMGB1) and the effects it has on the body. HMGB1 is one of the most prevalent RAGE's, as near as I can tell. It comes up in more studies...

- ***"HMGB1 ACTIVATES PROINFLAMMATORY SIGNALING VIA TLR5 LEADING TO ALLODYNIA"***

"Infectious and sterile inflammatory diseases are correlated with increased levels of high mobility group box 1 (HMGB1) in tissues and serum. Extracellular HMGB1 is known to activate Toll-like receptors (TLRs) 2 and 4 and RAGE (receptor for advanced glycation end products) in inflammatory conditions. Here, we find that TLR5 is also an HMGB1 receptor that was previously overlooked due to lack of functional expression in the cell lines usually used for studying TLR signaling. HMGB1 binding to TLR5 initiates the activation of an NF-κB signaling pathway in a MyD88-dependent manner, resulting in pro-inflammatory cytokine production and pain enhancement in vivo. Biophysical and in vitro results highlight an essential role for the C-terminal tail region of HMGB1 in facilitating interactions with TLR5. These results suggest that HMGB1-modulated TLR5 signaling is responsible for pain hypersensitivity." Study Link

I see HMGB1 come up in almost all modern diseases. This must be the most popular RAGEs.

The proof that carb consumption also contributes to lung cancer is in the following report from Oct 18, 2016, also. The underlying cause is inflammation.

- ***THE SER82 RAGE VARIANT AFFECTS LUNG FUNCTION AND SERUM RAGE IN SMOKERS AND SRAGE PRODUCTION IN VITRO***

"Abstract

INTRODUCTION:

Genome-Wide Association Studies have identified associations between lung function measures and Chronic Obstructive Pulmonary Disease (COPD) and chromosome region 6p21 containing the gene for the Advanced Glycation End Product Receptor (AGER, encoding RAGE). We aimed to (i) characterize RAGE expression in the lung, (ii) identify AGER transcripts, (iii) ascertain if SNP rs2070600 (Gly82Ser C/T) is associated with

lung function and serum sRAGE levels and (iv) identify whether the Gly82Ser variant is functionally important in altering sRAGE levels in an airway epithelial cell model.
METHODS:

Immunohistochemistry was used to identify RAGE protein expression in 26 human tissues and qPCR was used to quantify AGER mRNA in lung cells. Gene expression array data was used to identify AGER expression during lung development in 38 fetal lung samples. RNA-Seq was used to identify AGER transcripts in lung cells. sRAGE levels were assessed in cells and patient serum by ELISA. BEAS2B-R1 cells were transfected to overexpress RAGE protein with either the Gly82 or Ser82 variant and sRAGE levels identified.
RESULTS:

Immunohistochemical assessment of 6 adult lung samples identified high RAGE expression in the alveoli of healthy adults and individuals with COPD. AGER/RAGE expression increased across developmental stages in the human fetal lung at both the mRNA (38 samples) and protein levels (20 samples). Extensive AGER splicing was identified. The rs2070600T (Ser82) allele is associated with higher FEV1, FEV1/FVC and lower serum sRAGE levels in UK smokers. Using an airway epithelium model overexpressing the Gly82 or Ser82 variants we found that HMGB1 activation of the RAGE-Ser82 receptor results in lower sRAGE production.
CONCLUSIONS:
This study provides new information regarding the expression profile and potential role of RAGE in the human lung and shows a functional role of the Gly82Ser variant. These findings advance our understanding of the potential mechanisms underlying COPD particularly for carriers of this AGER polymorphism." STUDY LINK
I wonder if the ACS, American Cancer Society will take this information and realize what foods are responsible for this report showing how RAGEs have a role in COPD and ultimately lung cancer? Will it provoke a response from the ACS on the consumption of the foods responsible for this RAGE? Will they issue a warning or are they more concerned with an industry that depends on this disorder, the pharmaceutical industry, or maybe an industry that provokes this disorder, the grain industry?

You may ask though, shouldn't smoking play a larger role in this equation? I submit that if the glycation never existed in the first place, the smoking wouldn't play as large of a role as it does with the inflammation in the body. It takes the glycation to create the RAGE responsible for lung cancer, yet no one knows of glycation or its effects from the FDA, the USDA or the CDC. Who are they trying to protect? Why isn't glycation considered a disease?

In the following from an April 19, 2016, study, the emergence of the HMGB1

RAGE in head and the skin cancer, neck squamous cell carcinoma;

- *"CLINICAL VALUE OF HIGH MOBILITY GROUP BOX 1 AND THE RECEPTOR FOR ADVANCED GLYCATION END-PRODUCTS IN HEAD AND NECK CANCER: A SYSTEMATIC REVIEW"*

"Introduction   High mobility group box 1 is a versatile protein involved in gene transcription, extracellular signaling, and response to inflammation. Extracellularly, high mobility group box 1 binds to several receptors, notably the receptor for advanced glycation end-products. Expression of high mobility group box 1 and the receptor for advanced glycation end-products has been described in many cancers.

Objectives   To systematically review the available literature using PubMed and Web of Science to evaluate the clinical value of high mobility group box 1 and the receptor for advanced glycation end-products in head and neck squamous cell carcinomas.

Data Synthesis   A total of eleven studies were included in this review. High mobility group box 1 overexpression is associated with poor prognosis and many clinical and pathological characteristics of head and neck squamous cell carcinomas patients. Additionally, the receptor for advanced glycation end-products demonstrates potential value as a clinical indicator of tumor angiogenesis and advanced staging. In diagnosis, high mobility group box 1 demonstrates low sensitivity.

Conclusion   High mobility group box 1 and the receptor for advanced glycation end-products are associated with clinical and pathological characteristics of head and neck squamous cell carcinomas. Further investigation of the prognostic and diagnostic value of these molecules is warranted." Study Link

Although the study above was published in Oct 2016, this kind of evidence has been around for over 20 years. These reports started showing up in 1984;

Nonenzymatic *glycation* of human lens crystallin. Effect of aging and diabetes mellitus
We have examined the nonenzymatic glycation of human lens crystallin, an extremely long-lived protein, from 16 normal human ocular lenses 0.2-99 yr of age, and from 11 diabetic lenses 52-82-yr-old...the nonenzymatic glycation of nondiabetic lens crystallin may be regarded as a biological clock...The glucitol-lysine (Glc-Lys) content of soluble and insoluble crystallin was determined after reduction with H-borohydride followed by acid hydrolysis, boronic acid affinity chromatography, and high-pressure cation exchange chromatography...Over an age range comparable to that of the control samples, the diabetic crystallin samples contained about twice as much Glc-Lys.

More on cataracts is found later in this chapter. This study from Oct 6, 2016, shows glycations implication in cardiovascular disease;

- **"THERAPEUTIC INTERVENTIONS FOR ADVANCED GLYCATION-END PRODUCTS AND ITS RECEPTOR-MEDIATED CARDIOVASCULAR DISEASE"**

"Advanced glycation end products (AGEs) are a heterogeneous group of molecules formed from the non-enzymatic reaction of reducing sugars with the amino group of proteins, lipids, and nucleic acid. Interaction of AGEs with its cell-bound receptor (RAGE) results in the generation of oxygen radicals, nuclear factor kappa-β, pro-inflammatory cytokines and cell adhesion molecules, and is involved in the pathophysiology of cardiovascular diseases (CVD). Circulating soluble forms of RAGE (sRAGE) and endo-secretory RAGE (esRAGE) compete with RAGE for ligand binding and function as a decoy. This paper describes the endogenous and exogenous (high dietary AGEs, cooking food under high dry heat, elevated pH, and long period) sources of AGEs. AGE-RAGE-mediated CVD includes atherosclerosis, coronary artery disease, carotid artery disease, hypertension, peripheral vascular diseases, heart failure, cardiomyopathy, and microangiopathy. The therapeutic intervention with a reduction in AGEs and RAGE and elevation in sRAGE has been reported for the treatment of AGE-RAGE-mediated CVD. Reduction in levels of AGEs can be achieved by a reduction in consumption of food containing or creating the low amount of AGEs, cooking food at low temperature, moist heat, and shorter duration. AGE formation can be reduced with drugs, vitamins, and stoppage of cigarette smoking. Statins, telmisartan, and curcumin have been used for suppression of RAGE. Statins, ACE-inhibitors, Rosiglitazone and vitamin D have been used to increase levels of sRAGE. Finally, exogenous administration of sRAGE can be helpful in amelioration of CVD. In conclusion, AGE-RAGE-mediated CVD could be attenuated with a reduction in consumption of AGEs, suppression of RAGE and elevation of sRAGE."

Instead of looking at eliminating the glycating factor, their resolution to this problem is contained in more drugs. They think that creating more drugs to counteract the glycation is going to solve the problem of glycation. Is that because more drugs will ultimately lead to more drugs?

Statins are the most dangerous in the above equation as they unbalance your cholesterol which puts everything in your body out of balance. It's your cholesterol that regulates a good portion of your hormones. You should already know how much your hormones affect your emotions, energy, intelligence, aging, and basic proper functioning of your body, right down to digesting carbs (insulin). Granted insulin is made in the pancreas, although other more influential hormones are made in your fat which is what statins reduce.

Side effects of statins; *Common statin-related side effects (headaches,* *stomach upset, abnormal liver function tests and muscle cramps)... Side effects of statins include muscle pain, increased risk of diabetes mellitus, and abnormalities in liver enzyme tests. Additionally, they have rare but severe adverse effects, particularly muscle damage. As of 2010, a number of statins are on the market: atorvastatin, fluvastatin, lovastatin, pitavastatin, pravastatin, rosuvastatin, and simvastatin. Several combination preparations of a statin and another agent, such as ezetimibe/simvastatin, are also available. In 2005 sales were estimated at $18.7 billion in the United States.*

Side effects ultimately lead to other drugs down the road. It's inevitable. This is how the pharmaceutical corporations make as much money as they do. And you gladly give it to them, simply to keep up your addiction and later to fight your CVD or cancer. How much sense this make to you? What concerns me more than anything else is the fact the atorvastatin is the best selling pharmaceutical in history, with sales of $12.4 billion in 2008. With all of the side effects listed above, how many patients taking these drugs will not ever have to use any more pharmaceuticals. This is the way they guarantee a return consumer. I know. (I was one of them. I won't be anymore due to my keto diet.)

The best-selling statin is atorvastatin, which in 2003 became the best-selling pharmaceutical in history. The manufacturer Pfizer reported sales of US$12.4 billion in 2008. Pfizer and Monsanto were under one roof at in 2003. That was the year Pfizer started their divestiture of Monsanto. (Maybe it was the lawsuits that were starting to pile up, that they didn't appreciate.) I wonder how many lawsuits Pfizer has against itself for its pharmaceutical statins. Below are the contraindications for atorvastatin (Lipitor).

Contraindications
Active liver disease: cholestasis, hepatic encephalopathy, hepatitis, and jaundice
Unexplained elevations in AST or ALT levels
Pregnancy: Atorvastatin may cause fetal harm by affecting serum cholesterol and triglyceride levels, which are essential for fetal development.
Breastfeeding: Small amounts of other statin drugs have been found to pass into breast milk, although atorvastatin has not been studied, specifically.
Markedly elevated CPK levels or if a myopathy is suspected or diagnosed after dosing of atorvastatin has begun. Very rarely, atorvastatin may cause rhabdomyolysis, and it may be very serious leading to acute renal failure due to myoglobinuria. If rhabdomyolysis is suspected or diagnosed, atorvastatin therapy should be discontinued immediately. The likelihood of developing a myopathy is increased by the co-administration

of cyclosporine, fibric acid derivatives, erythromycin, niacin, and azole antifungals.

Adverse effects

Major

Diabetes mellitus type 2, an uncommon class effect of all statins. Myopathy with elevation of creatinine kinase (CK) and rhabdomyolysis are the most serious side effects, occurring rarely at a rate of 2.3 to 9.1 per 10,000 person-years among patients taking atorvastatin. As mentioned previously, atorvastatin should be discontinued immediately if this occurs. Persistent liver enzyme abnormalities occurred in 0.7% of patients who received atorvastatin in clinical trials. It is recommended that hepatic function be assessed with laboratory tests before beginning atorvastatin treatment and repeated as clinically indicated thereafter. If evidence of serious liver injury occurs while a patient is taking atorvastatin, it should be discontinued and not restarted until the etiology of the patient's liver dysfunction is defined. If no other cause is found, atorvastatin should be discontinued permanently.

Common

The following have been shown to occur in 1–10% of patients taking atorvastatin in clinical trials.

Arthralgia,

Diarrhea,

Dyspepsia,

Myalgia,

Nausea

High-dose atorvastatin has also been associated with worsening glycemic control.

Other

In 2014 the FDA reported memory loss, forgetfulness, and confusion with all statin products including atorvastatin. The symptoms were not serious, and they were rare and reversible on cessation of drug treatment.

Interactions

Interactions with clofibrate, fenofibrate, gemfibrozil, which are fibrates used in accessory therapy in many forms of hypercholesterolemia, usually in combination with statins, increase the risk of myopathy and rhabdomyolysis. Co-administration of atorvastatin with one of CYP3A4 inhibitors such as itraconazole, telithromycin, and voriconazole, may increase serum concentrations of atorvastatin, which may lead to adverse reactions. This is less likely to happen with other CYP3A4 inhibitors such as diltiazem, erythromycin, fluconazole, ketoconazole, clarithromycin, cyclos porine, protease inhibitors, or verapamil, and only rarely with other CYP3A4 inhibitors, such as amiodarone and aprepitant. Often, bosentan, fosphenytoin, and phenytoin, which are CYP3A4 inducers, can decrease the plasma concentrations of atorvastatin. Only rarely, though, barbiturates, carbamazepine, efavirenz, nevirapine, oxcarbazepine, r ifampin, and rifamycin, which are also CYP3A4 inducers, can decrease the plasma concentrations of atorvastatin. Oral contraceptives increased AUC values for norethisterone and ethinylestradiol; these increases should be

considered when selecting an oral contraceptive for a woman taking
atorvastatin.
Antacids can rarely decrease the plasma concentrations of statin drugs, but
do not affect the LDL-C-lowering efficacy.
Niacin also is proved to increase the risk of myopathy or rhabdomyolysis.
Statins may also alter the concentrations of other drugs, such
as warfarin or digoxin, leading to alterations in effect or a requirement for
clinical monitoring.
Vitamin D supplementation lowers atorvastatin and active metabolite
concentrations, yet synergistically reduces LDL and
total cholesterol concentrations. Grapefruit juice components are known
inhibitors of intestinal CYP3A4.
Co-administration of grapefruit juice with atorvastatin may cause an increase
in Cmax and AUC, which can lead to adverse reactions or overdose toxicity.
A few cases of myopathy have been reported when atorvastatin is given
with colchicine.

These are side effects of *Lipitor* and they include diarrhea, dyspepsia, myalgia, and nausea. Are you on statins? Did you read over your drug disclosure before you administered your dose? Do you fully know what this drug is doing to your body?

More importantly, were you told that you could cure this without drugs? Were you ever told that this disorder started with your diet of carbs? The earliest report in PMC I found was dated Jan 1974 and simply stated that weight reduction was important to controlling hyperlipoproteinemia, a fancy word for high amounts of apolipoproteins in the body which indicate levels of cholesterol. The apolipoprotein that's the most dangerous is apolipoprotein B. That's the one you get from carbs. This one is behind more disease than any of the other apolipoproteins.

With apolipoprotein B, an LDL particle being involved in more disorders than any of the other apolipoproteins, and apo α being the basis of HDL particles why isn't more attention devoted to balancing cholesterol than just lowering it? Were you aware that balancing your cholesterol was much more important to your body than lowering it? Lowering cholesterol is dangerous for the body as it's cholesterol that regulates your hormones, creates vitamin D in your skin to help usher in the LDL particles into your cells to use as fuel. Without the vitamin D, your cells couldn't operate properly and your LDL particles would build up in your bloodstream, waiting to be glycated or used as fuel, whichever comes first.

According to a study completed in 1995; *Population studies linking low*
cholesterol to noncoronary mortalities do not demonstrate cause-and-effect
relations. In fact, based on current studies, the opposite is more likely to be
the case. Drug intervention, however, should be used conservatively,

particularly in young adults and the elderly. Drugs should be used only after diet and lifestyle interventions have failed. The evidence linking high blood cholesterol to coronary atherosclerosis and cholesterol-lowering to its prevention is broad-based and definitive. Concerns about cholesterol lowering and spontaneously low cholesterols should be pursued but should not interfere with the implementation of current public policies to reduce the still heavy burden of atherosclerosis in Western society.

Another study from 1994 showed the rethinking of the low-fat hi-carb diet that has been pushed for over 40 years (probably at the insistence of Monsanto). Since they owned GD Searle at the time it makes me wonder, was it their intent to hook us on more drugs? Even as recent Dec 31, 2016, the dept. of research at Kaiser Permanente Southern California, Pasadena came to this conclusion;

From PMC, I found this report submitted Jun 17, 2013. It details the danger

of statin use;

- ### Statins in heart failure: do we need another trial?

Two recent large randomized controlled trials, however, appear to suggest statins do not have beneficial effects on heart failure. In addition to lowering cholesterol, statins are believed to have many pleiotropic effects which could possibly influence the pathophysiology of heart failure. (Pleiotropic – one cause for many diseases)
Further, hyperuricemia is frequently present in chronic HF and has been attributed to increased production or decreased urinary excretion of uric acid (UA) or both in a compromised circulation.135 An elevated plasma level of UA is linked with a wide variety of injurious processes comprising increased inflammatory markers, cell apoptosis, and ED,139 which could cumulatively worsen HF. Serum UA is known to be a marker of HF prognosis and mortality140–142 and statins have been shown to decrease UA levels by increasing urate excretion.143,144

Our medical industry has had research for over 20 years on the benefits of cholesterol and the dangers of lowering it, yet because of our dependence on grains and sugar and Monsanto's influence in the FDA and USDA, the recommendations from the USDA's agency for food labeling to food safety to *MyPlate, the CCNP* and at least 3 other agencies in the USDA alone, the CDC, the ADA, the ACS still recommend that you keep whole grains in your diet, regardless of the studies completed that show their danger. Why?

Monsanto is in the crop seed industry owning over 15 crop seed companies, all wanting to sell GMO seed, ready to handle Roundup herbicide to farmers contracted by Monsanto waiting to plant their next crop. They'll spray their crops according to their contract with Monsanto. It then goes on your table. Could Monsanto's old execs in the offices and agencies of the USDA and the FDA have anything to do with their decisions to ignore these facts? Or is this influence from Pfizer and Pharmacia? (I'm sure Monsanto stock is still in their portfolios.)

This article appeared 22 years ago in PubMed in Aug 1994. Even then low cholesterol was being questioned, yet in some corners, it's still promoted today;

- ***The questionable wisdom of a low-fat diet and cholesterol reduction***

Although hypercholesterolemia is associated with increased liability to death from heart disease, it is as frequently associated with increased overall life expectancy as with decreased life expectancy. These findings are incompatible with labeling hypercholesterolemia an overall health hazard. Moreover, it is questionable if the cardiovascular liability associated with hypercholesterolemia is either causal or reversible. The complex relationships between diet, serum cholesterol, atherosclerosis, and mortality and their interactions with genetic and environmental factors suggest that the effects of simple dietary prescriptions are unlikely to be predictable, let alone beneficial. These cautions are borne out by numerous studies which have shown that multifactorial primary intervention to lower cholesterol levels is as likely to increase death from cardiovascular causes as to decrease it. Importantly, the only significant overall effect of a cholesterol-lowering intervention that has ever been shown is increased mortality.

With Monsanto's influence in the FDA, the USDA, the EPA and who knows what else, who's to protect our food supply? You have to protect yourself. Monsanto has proven they can't self-regulate their industry and keep us safe. The best way to start being safe is to not eat their food, which happens to include all grains. If you don't buy them, that may send the message.

More evidence, published Dec 18, 2016, of its influence in cancer is when this HMGB1 RAGE rears its ugly head again;

- ***"BLOCKADE OF HIGH MOBILITY GROUP BOX 1 (HMGB1) AUGMENTS ANTI-TUMOR T-CELL RESPONSE INDUCED BY PEPTIDE VACCINATION AS A CO-ADJUVANT"***

"High Mobility Group Box 1 (HMGB1) is a member of the damage-associated molecular patterns (DAMPs), which cause inflammation and trigger innate immunity through Toll-like receptors (TLRs) 2/4 and the receptor for

advanced glycation end products (RAGE). We examined the effect of glycyrrhizin, a selective inhibitor of HMGB1, on the induction of cytotoxic T-lymphocytes (CTLs) in mice. B6 mice, either OT-1 spleen cell-transferred or untransferred, were immunized with an s.c. injection of the OVA257-264 peptide with topical imiquimod and glycyrrhizin was mixed with the antigen peptide. The proliferation of OT-1 cells after immunization was enhanced by glycyrrhizin. The effect of glycyrrhizin was confirmed in other adjuvant systems, such as CpG oligonucleotide and monophosphoryl lipid A (MPL), but glycyrrhizin was not effective in Freund's incomplete adjuvant system. The augmenting effects of glycyrrhizin were also observed in other synthetic HMGB1 inhibitors, i.e., gabexate mesylate, nafamostat, and sivelestat. Thus the effects are common to the HMGB1 inhibitors. Induction of CTLs detected by IFN-γ ELISPOT assay was similarly augmented by glycyrrhizin. In a therapeutic vaccine model, glycyrrhizin inhibited the growth of s.c. transplanted EG.7 tumors. Expression of inflammatory cytokines in the skin inoculation site was downregulated by glycyrrhizin. These results suggest that HMGB1 inhibitors might be useful as a co-adjuvant for peptide vaccination with an innate immunity receptor-related adjuvant. This article is protected by copyright. All rights reserved." Study Link

Were you ever told that this could happen if you continued your diet of bread, corn, soy and other carbs? (Neither was I.)

This is evidence of glycation's effect on the kidneys from this report dated Oct 6, 2016:

- **"AGES/SRAGE, A NOVEL RISK FACTOR IN THE PATHOGENESIS OF END-STAGE RENAL DISEASE"**

"Interaction of advanced glycation end products (AGEs) with its cell-bound receptor (RAGE) results in cell dysfunction through activation of nuclear factor kappa-B, increase in expression and release of inflammatory cytokines, and generation of oxygen radicals. Circulating soluble receptors, soluble receptor (sRAGE), endogenous secretory receptor (esRAGE) and cleaved receptor (cRGAE) act as a decoy for RAGE ligands and thus have cytoprotective effects. Low levels of sRAGE and esRAGE have been proposed as biomarkers for many diseases. However sRAGE and esRAGE levels are elevated in diabetes and chronic renal diseases and still, tissue injury occurs. It is possible that increases in levels of AGEs are greater than increases in the levels of soluble receptors in these two diseases. Some new parameters have to be used which could be universal biomarkers for cell dysfunction. It is hypothesized that increases in serum levels of AGEs are greater than the increases in the soluble receptors, and that the levels of AGEs is correlated with soluble receptors and that the ratios of AGEs/sRAGE, AGEs/esRAGE, and AGEs/cRAGE are elevated in patients with end-stage renal disease (ESRD) and would serve as a universal risk marker for ESRD. The study subject comprised of 88 patients with ESRD and 20 healthy controls. AGEs, sRAGE and esRAGE were measured using commercially available enzyme-linked immune assay kits. cRAGE was calculated by subtracting esRAGE from sRAGE. The data show that the

serum levels of AGEs, sRAGE, cRAGE are elevated and that the elevation of AGEs was greater than those of soluble receptors. The ratios of AGEs/sRAGE, AGEs/esRAGE, and AGEs/cRAGE were elevated and the elevation was similar in AGEs/sRAGE and AGEs/cRAGE but greater than AGEs/esRAGE. The sensitivity, specificity, accuracy, and positive and negative predictive value of AGEs/sRAGE and AGEs/cRAGE were 86.36 and 84.88%, 86.36 and 80.95%, 0.98 and 0.905, 96.2 and 94.8%, and 61.29 and 56.67% respectively. There was a positive correlation of sRAGE with esRAGE and cRAGE, and AGEs with esRAGE; and a negative correlation between sRAGE and AGEs/sRAGE, esRAGE and AGES/esRAGE, and cRAGE and AGES/cRAGE. In conclusion, AGEs/sRAGE, AGEs/cRAGE, and AGEs/esRAGE may serve as universal risk biomarkers for ESRD and that AGEs/sRAGE and AGEs/cRAGE are better risk biomarkers than AGEs/esRAGE." Study Link

This report from Sep15, 2016 is the evidence that breast cancer is influenced by glycation;

- *"INCREASED EXPRESSION OF THE RECEPTOR FOR ADVANCED LOCATION END-PRODUCTS (RAGE) IS ASSOCIATED WITH ADVANCED BREAST CANCER STAGE"*

"Abstract
BACKGROUND:
The receptor for advanced glycation end-products (RAGE) is a multiligand transmembrane receptor that is overexpressed in various pathological conditions including cancers. However, the expression pattern of RAGE in breast cancer tumors is still not completely clear.
METHODS:
In this study, we investigated the expression levels of RAGE in 25 fresh-frozen breast cancer samples and corresponding noncancerous tissue samples collected from breast cancer patients, by real-time polymerase chain reaction (PCR). Additionally, we performed immunohistochemistry on breast cancer specimens.
RESULTS:
The results indicate a high expression of the RAGE-encoding gene in the cancerous tissues. RAGE expression at the mRNA and protein levels was statistically significantly up-regulated in advanced-stage and triple-negative breast tumors and node-positive tissues compared with other tissues ($p <$ 0.001). A significant association between RAGE expression and tumor size was observed ($p = 0.029$).
CONCLUSIONS:
Overexpression of RAGE in advanced-stage tumors may be a useful biomarker for diagnosis and the prediction of breast cancer progression." Study Link

I'm only sorry that I could include studies and reports for all forms of cancer, but with they're being so many of them, that's a virtually impossible task.

I'll bet you didn't realize that your bone mineral density was a result of your diet, did you? (Nobody does.) Evidence of bone density decline from glycation is in this report from Dec14, 2016;

- *"ADVANCED GLYCATION END PRODUCTS, DIABETES, AND BONE STRENGTH"*

"Diabetic patients have a higher fracture risk than expected by their bone mineral density (BMD). Poor bone quality is the most suitable and explainable cause of the elevated fracture risk in this population. Advanced glycation end products (AGEs), which are diverse compounds generated via a non-enzymatic reaction between reducing sugars and amine residues, physically affect the properties of the bone material, one of a component of bone quality, through their accumulation in the bone collagen fibers. On the other hand, these compounds biologically act as agonists for these receptors for AGEs (RAGE) and suppress bone metabolism. The concentrations of AGEs and endogenous secretory RAGE, which acts as a "decoy receptor" that inhibits the AGEs-RAGE signaling axis, are associated with fracture risk in a BMD-independent manner. AGEs are closely associated with the pathogenesis of this unique clinical manifestation through physical and biological mechanisms in patients with diabetes mellitus." Study link

Evidence of Alzheimer's disease from glycation in this report from Oct 4, 2016;

"Genetic association between RAGE polymorphisms and Alzheimer's disease and Lewy body dementias in a Japanese cohort: a case-control study"

*"Abstract
BACKGROUND/AIMS:
Interaction of receptor for advanced glycation end products (RAGE) with amyloid-β increases amplification of oxidative stress and plays pathological roles in Alzheimer's disease (AD). Oxidative stress leads to α-synuclein aggregation and is also a major contributing factor in the pathogenesis of Lewy body dementias (LBDs). Therefore, we aimed to investigate whether RAGE gene polymorphisms were associated with AD and LBDs.
METHODS:
Four single nucleotide polymorphisms (SNPs)-rs1800624, rs1800625, rs184003, and rs2070600-of the gene were analyzed using a case-control study design comprising 288 AD patients, 76 LBDs patients, and 105 age-matched controls.
RESULTS:
Linkage disequilibrium (LD) examination showed strong LD from rs1800624 to rs2070600 on the gene (1.1 kb) in our cases in Japan. Rs184003 was associated with an increased risk of the AD. Although there were no statistical associations for the other three SNPs, haplotypic analyses detected genetic associations between AD and the RAGE gene. Although*

*relatively few cases were studied, results from the SNPs showed that they
did not modify the risk of developing LBDs in the Japanese population.
CONCLUSION: Our findings suggested that polymorphisms in the RAGE
gene are involved in genetic susceptibility to the AD. Copyright © 2016 John
Wiley & Sons, Ltd." Study Link*

With the above evidence showing its involvement in brain diseases, how
long will it take for this information to show up in the media? Doesn't anyone
of authority examine these reports? More evidence below of cancer-causing
agents from glycation leaving me to wonder; is anyone looking out for our
benefit? This next report is from Oct 3, 2016;

- **"M2 MACROPHAGES DO NOT FLY INTO A "RAGE"**

*"Tumor-associated macrophages (TAMs) are key elements in orchestrating
host responses inside tumor stroma. This population may undergo a
polarized activation process, thus rendering a heterogeneous spectrum of
phenotypes, where the classically activated type 1 macrophages (M1) and
the alternative activated type 2 macrophages (M2) represent two extreme
phenotypes. In this commentary, based on very recent research findings, we
intend to highlight how complex could be the crosstalk among all
components of tumor stroma, where the coexistence of non-natural partners
may even skew the canonical responses that we can expect." Study Link*

This is where your addiction starts with this evidence of glycation causing
agents in baby food. This is indicative of the glucose in the formula. Ask
yourself why this is done if glucose is capable of doing this much harm;

- **"PROTEIN BREAKDOWN AND RELEASE OF B-CASOMORPHINS
  DURING IN VITRO GASTRO-INTESTINAL DIGESTION OF
  STERILIZED MODEL SYSTEMS OF LIQUID INFANT FORMULA"**

*"Protein modifications occurring during sterilization of infant formulas can
affect protein digestibility and release of bioactive peptides. The effect
of glycation and cross-linking on protein breakdown and release of β-
casomorphins was evaluated during in vitro gastrointestinal digestion (GID)
of six sterilized model systems of infant formula. Protein degradation during
in vitro GID was evaluated by SDS-PAGE and by measuring the nitrogen
content of ultrafiltration (3kDa) permeates before and after in vitro GID of
model IFs. Glycation strongly hindered protein breakdown, whereas cross-
linking resulting from β-elimination reactions had a negligible effect. Only β-
casomorphin 7 (β-CM7) was detected (0.187-0.858mgL(-1)) at the end of the
intestinal digestion in all untreated IF model systems. The level of β-CM7 in
the sterilized model systems prepared without addition of sugars ranged
from 0.256 to 0.655mgL(-1). The release of this peptide during GID was
hindered by protein glycation." Study Link*

Here's your proof that glucose and its glycative results are responsible for
type 1 diabetes (the one thought to be an autoimmune disorder), this was
just released Oct15, 2016. Watch to see if you'll hear anything about it. If you
don't, it's probably because Big Pharma has something to say about it;

- **"THE RECEPTOR FOR ADVANCED GLYCATION ENDPRODUCTS DRIVES T CELL SURVIVAL AND INFLAMMATION IN TYPE 1 DIABETES MELLITUS"**

"The ways in which environmental factors participate in the progression of autoimmune diseases are not known. After initiation, it takes years before hyperglycemia develops in patients at risk for type 1 diabetes (T1D). The receptor for advanced glycation endproducts (RAGE) is a scavenger receptor of the Ig family that binds damage-associated molecular patterns and advanced glycated endproducts and can trigger cell activation. We previously found constitutive intracellular RAGE expression in lymphocytes from patients with T1D. In this article, we show that there is increased RAGE expression in T cells from at-risk euglycemic relatives who progress to T1D compared with healthy control subjects, and in the CD8+ T cells in the at-risk relatives who do versus those who do not progress to T1D. Detectable levels of the RAGE ligand high mobility group box 1 were present in serum from at-risk subjects and patients with T1D. Transcriptome analysis of RAGE+ versus RAGE- T cells from patients with T1D showed differences in signaling pathways associated with increased cell activation and survival. Additional markers for effector memory cells and inflammatory function were elevated in the RAGE+ CD8+ cells of T1D patients and at-risk relatives of patients before disease onset. These studies suggest that expression of RAGE in T cells of subjects progressing to disease predates dysglycemia. These findings imply that RAGE expression enhances the inflammatory function of T cells, and its increased levels observed in T1D patients may account for the chronic autoimmune response when damage-associated molecular patterns are released after cell injury and killing."
STUDY LINK

Evidence of the role of AGEs in the process of neurodegenerative diseases in this study from Sep 21, 2016;

- **"IMPACT OF NON-ENZYMATIC GLYCATION IN NEURODEGENERATIVE DISEASES: ROLE OF NATURAL PRODUCTS IN PREVENTION"**

"Non-enzymatic protein glycosylation is the addition of free carbonyls to the free amino groups of proteins, amino acids, lipoproteins and nucleic acids resulting in the formation of early glycation products. The early glycation products are also known as Maillard reaction which undergoes dehydration, cyclization, and rearrangement to form advanced glycation end-products (AGEs). By and large, the researchers in the past have also established that glycation and the AGEs are responsible for the most type of metabolic disorders, including diabetes mellitus, cancer, neurological disorders and aging. The amassing of AGEs in the tissues of neurodegenerative diseases shows its involvement in diseases. Therefore, it is likely that inhibition of glycation reaction may extend the lifespan of an individual. The hunt for inhibitors of glycation, mainly using in vitro models, has identified natural compounds able to prevent glycation, especially

polyphenols and other natural antioxidants. Extrapolation of results of in vitro studies on the in vivo situation is not straightforward due to differences in the conditions and mechanism of glycation, and bioavailability problems. Nevertheless, existing data allow postulating that enrichment of diet in natural anti-glycating agents may attenuate glycation and, in consequence, may halt the aging and neurological problems." Study Link

How long will it take for this information to be publicized? If it isn't, why not? Is it because there's no money in it?

The following is evidence of glycations role in cardiovascular disease from Sep 16, 2016;

- *"ADVANCED GLYCATION END-PRODUCTS INDUCE APOPTOSIS OF VASCULAR SMOOTH MUSCLE CELLS: A MECHANISM FOR VASCULAR CALCIFICATION"*

"Vascular calcification, especially medial artery calcification, is associated with cardiovascular death in patients with diabetes mellitus and chronic kidney disease (CKD). To determine the underlying mechanism of vascular calcification, we have demonstrated in our previous report that advanced glycation end-products (AGEs) stimulated calcium deposition in vascular smooth muscle cells (VSMCs) through excessive oxidative stress and phenotypic transition into osteoblastic cells. Since AGEs can induce apoptosis, in this study we investigated its role on VSMC apoptosis, focusing mainly on the underlying mechanisms. A rat VSMC line (A7r5) was cultured and treated with glycolaldehyde-derived AGE-bovine serum albumin (AGE3-BSA). Apoptotic cells were identified by Terminal deoxynucleotidyl transferase UTP nick end labeling (TUNEL) staining. To quantify apoptosis, an enzyme-linked immunosorbent assay (ELISA) for histone-complexed DNA fragments was employed. Real-time PCR was performed to determine the mRNA levels. Treatment of A7r5 cells with AGE3-BSA from 100 µg/mL concentration markedly increased apoptosis, which was suppressed by Nox inhibitors. AGE3-BSA significantly increased the mRNA expression of NAD (P)H oxidase components including Nox4 and p22(phox), and these findings were confirmed by protein levels using immunofluorescence. The dihydroethidium assay showed that compared with BSA, AGE3-BSA increased reactive oxygen species level in A7r5 cells. Furthermore, AGE3-induced apoptosis was significantly inhibited by siRNA-mediated knockdown of Nox4 or p22 (phox). Double knockdown of Nox4 and p22 (phox) showed a similar inhibitory effect on apoptosis as single gene silencing. Thus, our results demonstrated that NAD (P)H oxidase-derived oxidative stress is involved in AGEs-induced apoptosis of VSMCs. These findings might be important to understand the pathogenesis of vascular calcification in diabetes and CKD."

Evidence of glycation from this study completed last year on mental disorders like schizophrenia;

- **"THE REGULATION OF SOLUBLE RECEPTOR FOR AGES CONTRIBUTES TO CARBONYL STRESS IN SCHIZOPHRENIA"**

"Our previous study showed that enhanced carbonyl stress is closely related to schizophrenia. The endogenous secretory receptor for advanced glycation end-products (esRAGE) is a splice variant of the AGER gene and is one of the soluble forms of RAGE. esRAGE is considered to be a key molecule for alleviating the burden of carbonyl stress by entrapping advanced glycation end-products (AGEs). In the current study, we conducted genetic association analyses focusing on AGER, in which we compared 212 schizophrenic patients to 214 control subjects. We also compared esRAGE levels among a subgroup of 104 patients and 89 controls and further carried out measurements of total circulating soluble RAGE (sRAGE) in 25 patients and 49 healthy subjects. Although the genetic association study yielded inconclusive results, multiple regression analysis indicated that a specific haplotype composed of rs17846798, rs2071288, and a 63 bp deletion, which were in perfect linkage disequilibrium (r2 = 1), and rs2070600 (Gly82Ser) were significantly associated with a marked decrease in serum esRAGE levels. Furthermore, compared to healthy subjects, schizophrenia showed significantly lower esRAGE (p = 0.007) and sRAGE (p = 0.03) levels, respectively. This is the first study to show that serum esRAGE levels are regulated by a newly identified specific haplotype in AGER and that a subpopulation of schizophrenic patients is more vulnerable to carbonyl stress. Copyright © 2016 The Authors. Published by Elsevier Inc. All rights reserved."* Study Link

Methylglyoxal is what makes up pyruvic acid which is a foundation for energy expenditure. It comes from glycogen which comes from glucose and can be made into lipids to be used for cholesterol or glucose to be used by your brain when the ketones aren't enough to power all lobes in the brain. This the link from glucose to disease through its conversion to AGEs, advanced glycation endproducts as explained by this study published Sep 2016;

- **"Methylglyoxal in Metabolic Disorders: Facts, Myths, and Promises"**

"Glucose and fructose metabolism originates the highly reactive by-product methylglyoxal (MG), which is a strong precursor of advanced glycation end products (AGE). The MG has been implicated in classical diabetic complications such as retinopathy, nephropathy, and neuropathy, but has also been recently associated with cardiovascular diseases and central nervous system disorders such as cerebrovascular diseases and dementia. Recent studies even suggested its involvement in insulin resistance and beta-cell dysfunction, contributing to the early development of type2 diabetes and creating a vicious circle between glycation and hyperglycemia. Despite several drugs and natural compounds have been identified in the last years in order to scavenge MG and inhibit AGE formation, we are still far from having an effective strategy to prevent MG-induced mechanisms. This review summarizes the endogenous and exogenous sources of MG, also addressing the current controversy about the importance of exogenous MG

sources. The mechanisms by which MG changes cell behavior and its involvement in type2 diabetes development and complications and the pathophysiological implication are also summarized. Particular emphasis will be given to the pathophysiological relevance of studies using higher MG doses, which may have produced biased results. Finally, we also overview the current knowledge about detoxification strategies, including modulation of endogenous enzymatic systems and exogenous compounds able to inhibit MG effects on biological systems." Study Link

Evidence of glycations influence in pancreatic complications was detailed in this report dated Aug 22, 2016;

- **"ADVANCED GLYCATION END PRODUCTS IMPAIR GLUCOSE-STIMULATED INSULIN SECRETION OF A PANCREATIC B-CELL LINE INS-1-3 BY DISTURBANCE OF MICROTUBULE CYTOSKELETON VIA P38/MAPK ACTIVATION"**

Advanced glycation end products (AGEs) are believed to be involved in diverse complications of diabetes mellitus. Overexposure to AGEs of pancreatic β-cells leads to decreased insulin secretion and cell apoptosis. Here, to understand the cytotoxicity of AGEs to pancreatic β-cells, we used INS-1-3 cells as a β-cell model to address this question, which was a subclone of INS-1 cells and exhibited a high level of insulin expression and high sensitivity to glucose stimulation. Exposed to a large dose of AGEs, even though more insulin was synthesized, its secretion was significantly reduced from INS-1-3 cells. Further, AGEs treatment led to a time-dependent increase of depolymerized microtubules, which was accompanied by an increase of activated p38/MAPK in INS-1-3 cells. Pharmacological inhibition of p38/MAPK by SB202190 reversed microtubule depolymerization to a stabilized polymerization status but could not rescue the reduction of insulin release caused by AGEs. Taken together, these results suggest a novel role of AGEs-induced impairment of insulin secretion, which is partially due to a disturbance of microtubule dynamics that resulted from an activation of the p38/MAPK pathway." Study Link

In my estimation, this is the worst manifestation of bread in the diet. Amyloid plaque is at the root of most modern diseases, ranging from cancer to heart disease to arthritis to Alzheimer's disease and Parkinson's disease. This report is from Aug22, 2016;

- **"GLYCATION INDUCED GENERATION OF AMYLOID FIBRIL STRUCTURES BY GLUCOSE METABOLITES"**

"The non-enzymatic reaction (glycation) of reducing sugars with proteins has received increased interest in dietary and therapeutic research lately. In the present work, the impact of glycation on structural alterations of camel serum albumin (CSA) by different glucose metabolites was studied. Glycation of CSA was evaluated by specific fluorescence of advanced glycation end-products (AGEs) and determination of available amino groups. Further, conformational changes in CSA during glycation were also studied using 8-analino 1-naphthalene sulfonic acid (ANS) binding assay, circular dichroism

(CD) and thermal analysis. Intrinsic fluorescence measurement of CSA showed a 22 nm red shift after methylglyoxal treatment, suggesting glycation induced denaturation of CSA. Rayleigh scattering analysis showed glycation induced turbidity and aggregation in CSA. Furthermore, ANS binding to native and glycated-CSA reflected perturbation in the environment of hydrophobic residues. However, CD spectra did not reveal any significant modifications in the secondary structure of the glycated-CSA. Thioflavin T (ThT) fluorescence of CSA increased after glycation, illustrated cross β-structure and amyloid formation. Transmission electron microscopy (TEM) analysis further reaffirms the formation of aggregate and amyloid. In summary, glucose metabolites induced conformational changes in CSA and produced aggregate and amyloid structures."

This is more evidence of glycation's involvement in Alzheimer's disease. This report was submitted on Aug 24, 2016, have you heard anything about this yet? Who doesn't want you to know? Who have interests in selling your medication for memory loss? How would you learn this information if you didn't see it here? Do you know where to look for it? Do you even know to look for it? Am I fishing or can this be a conspiracy?

- ***"HMGB1 AND THROMBIN MEDIATE THE BLOOD-BRAIN BARRIER DYSFUNCTION ACTING AS BIOMARKERS OF NEUROINFLAMMATION AND PROGRESSION TO NEURODEGENERATION IN ALZHEIMER'S DISEASE"***

"BACKGROUND:
The blood-brain barrier (BBB) dysfunction represents an early feature of Alzheimer's disease (AD) that precedes the hallmarks of amyloid beta (amyloid β) plaque deposition and neuronal neurofibrillary tangle (NFT) formation. A damaged BBB correlates directly with neuroinflammation involving microglial activation and reactive astrogliosis, which is associated with increased expression and/or release of high-mobility group box protein 1 (HMGB1) and thrombin. However, the link between the presence of these molecules, BBB damage, and progression to neurodegeneration in the AD is still elusive. Therefore, we aimed to profile and validate non-invasive clinical biomarkers of BBB dysfunction and neuroinflammation to assess the progression to neurodegeneration in mild cognitive impairment (MCI) and AD patients.
METHODS:
We determined the serum levels of various proinflammatory damage-associated molecules in aged control subjects and patients with MCI or AD using validated ELISA kits. We then assessed the specific and direct effects of such molecules on BBB integrity in vitro using human primary brain microvascular endothelial cells or a cell line.
RESULTS:
We observed a significant increase in serum HMGB1 and soluble receptor for advanced glycation end products (sRAGE) that correlated well with amyloid beta levels in AD patients (vs. control subjects). Interestingly, serum HMGB1 levels were significantly elevated in MCI patients compared to

controls or AD patients. In addition, as a marker of BBB damage, soluble thrombomodulin (TM) antigen, and activity were significantly (and distinctly) increased in MCI and AD patients. Direct in vitro BBB integrity assessment further revealed a significant and concentration-dependent increase in paracellular permeability to dextrans by HMGB1 or α-thrombin, possibly through disruption of zona occludins-1 bands. Pre-treatment with anti-HMGB1 monoclonal antibody blocked HMGB1 effects and leaving BBB integrity intact.
CONCLUSIONS:
Our current studies indicate that thrombin and HMGB1 are causal proximate proinflammatory mediators of BBB dysfunction, while STM levels may indicate BBB endothelial damage; HMGB1 and sRAGE might serve as clinical biomarkers for progression and/or therapeutic efficacy along the AD spectrum." Study Link

With the previous study being completed last year, I'm curious to learn how long it will take for this information to be publicized. (If it ever is.)

More evidence of the damaging effects of glycation was submitted July 15, 2016. Have you heard anything about this report yet?

"The false alarm hypothesis: Food allergy is associated with high dietary advanced glycation end-products and proglycating dietary sugars that mimic alarmins."
"The incidence of food allergy has increased dramatically in the last few decades in westernized developed countries. We propose that the Western lifestyle and diet promote innate danger signals and immune responses through production of "alarmins. Alarmins are endogenous molecules secreted from cells undergoing nonprogrammed cell death that signal tissue and cell damage. High molecular group S (HMGB1) is a major alarmin that binds to the receptor for advanced glycation end-products (RAGE). Advanced glycation end-products (AGEs) are also present in foods. We propose the "false alarm" hypothesis, in which AGEs that are present in or formed from the food in our diet are predisposing to food allergy. The Western diet is high in AGEs, which are derived from cooked meat, oils, and cheese. AGEs are also formed in the presence of a high concentration of sugars. We propose that a diet high in AGEs and AGE-forming sugars results in misinterpretation of a threat from dietary allergens, promoting the development of food allergy. AGEs and other alarmins inadvertently prime innate signaling through multiple mechanisms, resulting in the development of allergic phenotypes. Current hypotheses and models of food allergy do not adequately explain the dramatic increase in food allergy in Western countries. Dietary AGEs and AGE-forming sugars might be the missing link, a hypothesis supported by a number of convincing epidemiologic and experimental observations, as discussed in this article." Study Link
Again no alert about this evidence of the influence of glycation in dementia submitted in Aug 2016 from the Oxford Journal of Gerontology;

- *"INFLAMMATORY BIOMARKERS PREDICT DOMAIN-SPECIFIC COGNITIVE DECLINE IN OLDER ADULTS"*

"BACKGROUND:
Vascular risk factors, including inflammation, may contribute to dementia development. We investigated the associations between peripheral inflammatory biomarkers and cognitive decline in five domains (memory, construction, language, psychomotor speed, and executive function).

METHODS:
Community-dwelling older adults from the Ginkgo Evaluation of Memory Study (n = 1,159, aged 75 or older) free of dementia at baseline were included and followed for up to 7 years. Ten biomarkers were measured at baseline representing different sources of inflammation: vascular inflammation (pentraxin 3 and serum amyloid P), endothelial function (endothelin-1), metabolic function (adiponectin, resistin, and plasminogen activating inhibitor-1), oxidative stress (receptor for advanced glycation end products), and general inflammation (interleukin-6, interleukin-2, and interleukin-10). A combined z-score was created from these biomarkers to represent total inflammation across these sources. We utilized generalized estimating equations that included an interaction term between z-scores and time to assess the effect of inflammation on cognitive decline, adjusting for demographics (such as age, race/ethnicity, and sex), cardiovascular risk factors, and apolipoprotein E ε4 carrier status. A Bonferroni-adjusted significance level of .01 was used. We explored associations between individual biomarkers and cognitive decline without adjustment for multiplicity.

RESULTS:
The combined inflammation z-score was significantly associated with memory and psychomotor speed (p < .01). Pentraxin 3, serum amyloid P, endothelin-1, and interleukin-2 were associated with a change in at least one cognitive domain (p < .05).

CONCLUSION:
Our results suggest that total inflammation is associated with memory and psychomotor speed. In particular, systemic inflammation, vascular inflammation, and altered endothelial function may play roles in the domain-specific cognitive decline of nondemented individuals. © The Author 2016. Published by Oxford University Press on behalf of The Gerontological Society of America. All rights reserved."   Study Link

Are you beginning to wonder why we've never been informed of these dangers? Evidence below of glycation in lung cancer was submitted on Aug 9, 2016. I've not heard anything about this. Doesn't the ACS care? They're still recommending carbs in the diet, so they must not;

"advanced glycation end-Products Enhance Lung Cancer Cell Invasion and Migration"

"Effects of carboxymethyl-lysine (CML) and pentosidine, two advanced glycation end-products (AGEs), upon invasion and migration in A549 and Calu-6 cells, two non-small cell lung cancer (NSCLC) cell lines were examined. CML or pentosidine at 1, 2, 4, 8 or 16 µmol/L were added into cells. Proliferation, invasion, and migration were measured. CML or pentosidine at 4-16 µmol/L promoted invasion and migration in both cell lines and increased the production of reactive oxygen species, tumor necrosis factor-α, interleukin-6 and transforming growth factor-β1. CML or pentosidine at 2-16 µmol/L up-regulated the protein expression of AGE receptor, p47(phox), intercellular adhesion molecule-1 and fibronectin in test NSCLC cells. Matrix metalloproteinase-2 protein expression in A549 and Calu-6 cells was increased by CML or pentosidine at 4-16 µmol/L. These two AGEs at 2-16 µmol/L enhanced nuclear factor κ-B (NF-κ B) p65 protein expression and p38 phosphorylation in A549 cells. However, CML or pentosidine at 4-16 µmol/L up-regulated NF-κB p65 and p-p38 protein expression in Calu-6 cells. These findings suggest that CML and pentosidine, by promoting the invasion, migration, and production of associated factors, benefit NSCLC metastasis." Study Link

This is the evidence of your back problems being caused by glycation. This study shows how the inflammatory responses to glycation causing vertebral disk degeneration;

- **"IL-1β/HMGB1 signaling promotes the inflammatory cytokines release via TLR signaling in human intervertebral disc cells"**

"Inflammation and cytokines have been recognized to correlate with intervertebral disc (IVD) degeneration (IDD), via mediating the development of clinical signs and symptoms. However, the regulation mechanism remains unclear. We aimed at investigating the regulatory role of interleukin (IL)β and high mobility group box 1 (HMGB1) in the inflammatory response in human IVD cells and then explored the signaling pathways mediating such regulatory effect. Firstly, the promotion of inflammatory cytokines in IVD cells was examined with ELISA method. And then western blot and real-time quantitative PCR were performed to analyze the expression of toll-like receptors (TLRs), receptors for advanced glycation endproducts (RAGE) and NF-κB signaling markers in the IL-1β- or (and) HMGB1-treated IVD cells. Results demonstrated that either IL-1β or HMGB1 promoted the release of the inflammatory cytokines such as prostaglandin E2 (PGE2), TNF-α, IL-6 and IL-8 in human IVD cells. And the expression of matrix metalloproteinases (MMPs) such as MMP-1, -3 and -9 was also additively up-regulated by IL-1β and HMGB1. We also found such additive promotion to the expression of TLR-2, TLR-4 and RAGE, and the NF-κB signaling in intervertebral disc cells. In summary, our study demonstrated that IL-1β and HMGB1 additively promote the release of inflammatory cytokines and the expression of MMPs in human IVD cells. The TLRs and RAGE and the NF-κB signaling were also additively promoted by IL-1β and HMGB1. Our study

implied that the additive promotion by IL-1β and HMGB1 to inflammatory cytokines and MMPs might aggravate the progression of IDD." Study Link

That study was submitted on Sep 16, 2016. I would have thought that I would have heard something about this by now, but I guess there's not enough money in curing. There's only enough money in treatment, as in continuous treatment.

It has to do with supply and demand. In this case, it's the pharmaceutical industry supplying its own demand...for customers, that is. They must think that the crop seed industry isn't sending them enough. If that isn't greed, I don't know what it.

Even unborn babies are not immune to the effects of what this industry is intent on putting as many Americans as they can, though. The damage they choose to ignore is in the glycation that's evidenced by this report dated Aug 10, 2016. How long do you think it will take for this information to be publicized? My estimate: never. (No money in it);

- **"ACCUMULATION OF ADVANCED GLYCATION END PRODUCTS INVOLVED IN INFLAMMATION AND CONTRIBUTING TO SEVERE PREECLAMPSIA, IN MATERNAL BLOOD, UMBILICAL BLOOD AND PLACENTAL TISSUES"**

Abstract
OBJECTIVE:
To investigate the expression of advanced glycation end products (AGEs) and the receptor for AGE (RAGEs) in maternal blood, umbilical blood and placental tissues in women with severe preeclampsia (PE) as well as any association with inflammatory processes.
METHODS:
The expressions of AGEs, RAGE, tumor necrosis factor-alpha (TNF)-α and vascular cell adhesion molecule-1 (VCAM)-1 in placental tissues were measured using immunohistochemistry. The levels of AGEs, RAGE, TNF-α and VCAM-1 in maternal blood, umbilical blood and placental extracts were assessed using enzyme-linked immunosorbent assays. Placental RAGE, TNF-α, and VCAM-1 mRNA expression levels were determined by PCR. Placental AGEs, RAGE, TNF-α and VCAM-1 protein levels were determined by western blotting.
RESULTS:
The levels of AGEs, TNF-α, and VCAM-1 in the maternal tissues and umbilical blood were significantly higher in the SPE group than in the normal pregnancy (NP) controls ($p < 0.05$). The serum level of sRAGE in the umbilical blood was lower in the SPE group than in the NP controls ($p < 0.05$), while sRAGE was higher in the maternal blood of SPE than in the NP ($p < 0.05$). The maternal serum levels of AGEs were positively correlated with that of TNF-α and VCAM-1 in the maternal blood. There were no

correlations between the levels of RAGE, TNF-α or VCAM-1 in maternal blood or umbilical serum. There were no correlations between the levels of sRAGE and TNF-α or VCAM-1 in maternal blood or umbilical serum. The levels of AGEs were positively correlated with those of TNF-α and VCAM-1 in placental lysates.
CONCLUSION:
AGEs and RAGE appear to act as important mediators in regulating the inflammatory pathways of preeclampsia.
From this report from Aug 9, 2016, ovarian cancer is a consequence of glycation;

- *S100B MEDIATES STEMNESS OF OVARIAN CANCER STEM-LIKE CELLS THROUGH INHIBITING P53*

"S100B is one of the members of the S100 protein family and is involved in the progression of a variety of cancers. Ovarian cancer is driven by cancer stem-like cells (CSLCs) that are involved in tumor genesis, metastasis, chemoresistance, and relapse. We then hypothesized that S100B might exert pro-tumor effects by regulating ovarian CSLCs stemness, a key characteristic of CSLCs. First, we observed the high expression of S100B in ovarian cancer specimens when compared to that in normal ovary. The S100B upregulation associated with more advanced tumor stages, poorer differentiation and poorer survival. In addition, elevated S100B expression correlated with increased expression of stem cell markers including CD133, Nanog, and Oct4. Then, we found that S100B was preferentially expressed in CD133+ ovarian CSLCs derived from both ovarian cancer cell lines and primary tumors of patients. More importantly, we revealed that S100B knockdown suppressed the in vitro self-renewal and in vivo tumorigenicity of ovarian CSLCs and decreased their expression of stem cell markers. S100B ectopic expression endowed non-CSLCs with stemness, which has been demonstrated with both in vitro and in vivo experiments. Mechanically, we demonstrated that the underlying mechanism of S100B-mediated effects on CSLCs stemness was not dependent on its binding with a receptor for advanced glycation end products (RAGE), but might be through intracellular regulation, through the inhibition of p53 expression and phosphorylation. In conclusion, our results elucidate the importance of S100B in the maintenance of ovarian CSLCs stemness, which might provide a promising therapeutic target for ovarian cancer. Stem Cells 2016." Study Link
HMGB1 is a label that's been assigned to a type of AGE or RAGE. Its importance lies in its ability to create pain in your body. This is one of over 11,851 warnings and notices of what glycation does to the body that available for your perusal on the effects of glycation on PubMed;

The Emerging Role of HMGB1 in Neuropathic Pain: A Potential Therapeutic Target for Neuroinflammation
Neuropathic pain (NPP) is the intolerable, persistent, and specific type of long-term pain. It is considered to be a direct consequence of pathological

changes affecting the somatosensory system and can be debilitating for affected patients. Despite recent progress and growing interest in understanding the pathogenesis of the disease, NPP still presents a major diagnostic and therapeutic challenge. High mobility group box 1 (HMGB1) mediates inflammatory and immune reactions in nervous system and emerging evidence reveals that HMGB1 plays an essential role in neuroinflammation through receptors such as Toll-like receptors (TLR), receptor for advanced glycation end products (RAGE), C-X-X motif chemokines receptor 4 (CXCR4), and N-methyl-D-aspartate (NMDA) receptor. In this review, we present evidence from studies that address the role of HMGB1 in NPP. First, we review studies aimed at determining the role of HMGB1 in NPP and discuss the possible mechanisms underlying HMGB1-mediated NPP progression where receptors for HMGB1 are involved. Then we review studies that address HMGB1 as a potential therapeutic target for NPP. Study Link

The following study was completed in July 2010, explaining the health benefits of calorie restriction. This is what was being researched over 120 years ago, as ketonuria was noticed in the urine of fasting patients, giving them ketonemia. This is a condition that best serves to heal in the body for multiple reasons and has been shown to heal many diseases, simply from fasting. Since 500BC fasting has been used to cure many diseases with astonishing success. This is what's known as ketosis today and is what your body goes through as a healing, fat burning type of metabolism. It uses your own fat to provide everything from hormones to glucose, through gluconeogenesis, the perfect glucose for the body as it made from your fat, making it a clean glucose source;

Dietary Interventions to Extend Life Span and Health Span Based on Calorie Restriction

The societal impact of obesity, diabetes, and other metabolic disorders continues to rise despite increasing evidence of their negative long-term consequences on health span, longevity, and aging. Unfortunately, dietary management and exercise frequently fail as remedies, underscoring the need for the development of alternative interventions to successfully treat metabolic disorders and enhance lifespan and health span. Using calorie restriction (CR)—which is well known to improve both health and longevity in controlled studies—as their benchmark, gerontologists are coming closer to identifying dietary and pharmacological therapies that may be applicable to aging humans. This review covers some of the more promising interventions targeted to affect pathways implicated in the aging process as well as variations on classical CR that may be better suited to human adaptation. Another report submitted Nov, 08 to the *Official Journal of the International League Against Epilepsy*, basically said the same thing while they were looking for the best way to approach putting the body into ketosis;

The ketogenic diet (KD) is a 90% fat diet that is an effective treatment for intractable epilepsy. Rapid initiation of the KD requires hospital admission because of the complexity of the protocol and frequent mild and moderate

adverse events. The purpose of the study was to compare the efficacy of a gradual KD initiation with the standard KD initiation preceded by a 24- to 48-h fast.

Perhaps the most damning report against aging was issued in January of 1984, yet nothing was mentioned about this report; it was one of the first indications of what glycation does to the body and with a major cause of glycation being glucose or sugar, I have to wonder why the FDA didn't say anything about it then. Why weren't we, at least, informed about this study? Industry concerns?

- ● *Collagen aging in vitro by nonenzymatic glycosylation and browning*

Aging and diabetes mellitus are associated with cross-linking and nonenzymatic glycosylation of collagen. Incubation of tendon fibers with reducing sugars results in increased breaking time in urea similar to that seen in aging, and in nonenzymatic glycosylation and browning. Effect of a sugar is proportional to the amount of sugar available in the open chain form. The increase in breaking time correlates with the appearance of chromophores characteristic of crosslinked browning products. Collagen altered by nonenzymatic browning may play a role in some age-like major complications of diabetes. Study Link

This evidence of glycation's role in atherosclerosis was in this study submitted in May 1988. Was this publicized? Did you hear about this? Did the FDA know?

Diminished adhesion of endothelial aortic cells on fibronectin and collagen layers after nonenzymatic glycation
Adhesion of bovine endothelial cells on fibronectin and collagen before and after nonenzymatic glycation in vitro has been studied.
Nonenzymatic glycation of these proteins reduced their ability to bind endothelial cells. Furthermore, nonenzymatically glycated fibronectin failed to bind to normal and nonenzymatically glycated gelatin and to fibrin. So gelatin and fibrin Sepharoses can be used to separate highly glycated fibronectins from fibronectins with a low degree of nonenzymatic glucose substitution. Sodium dodecyl sulfate-polyacrylamide gel electrophoresis did not demonstrate a covalent cross-link between nonenzymatically glycated fibronectins. These results present further evidence for the role of nonenzymatic glycation of proteins in the development of vascular complications in long-term diabetes and of atherosclerosis.   Study Link
This shows the damage done by glycation on the blood. I posted this study because I wanted to note what the first sentence states, that this damage, at the time of publication, had been known for 20 years. The date of this study

is marked on July 29, 1988. That means that his damage was discovered in 1968, 48 years ago.

Glycated haemoglobins

The association between elevated levels of glycated hemoglobins and diabetes mellitus has been known for twenty years [92]. Since then the determination of glycated hemoglobins has become a valuable tool for the objective assessment of long-term glycemia in diabetic patients. The marked clinical interest in reliable measurements of glycated hemoglobins has stimulated the development and perfection of the necessary methodology. Limitations of the techniques have led to an investigation of the underlying causes. Some of them led to the recognition of processes that were not known to occur in vivo before, such as glycation at sites other than the amino terminus of the beta-chains, modification of hemoglobin by reactants other than glucose or the existence of labile hemoglobin adducts. With ideal methodology, these features would have gone unnoticed. Furthermore, the determination of glycated hemoglobin in large populations of diabetic patients has to lead to the discovery of new, clinically silent mutant hemoglobins. Today, the routine determination of glycated hemoglobins in diabetic patients probably represents the broadest screening for mutant hemoglobins. The experience with glycated hemoglobins shows that overcoming difficulties in their determination, and progress in biomedical research, are closely intertwined.
This study shows how proteins exposed to glucose undergoes oxidative stress, the basis of aging;

"Autoxidative glycosylation": free radicals and glycation theory.
Studies have shown that glycation in vitro is complicated by the ability of glucose to oxidize, in the presence of trace amounts of a transition metal, generating protein-reactive ketoaldehydes, hydrogen peroxide, and diverse free radicals. Protein exposed to glucose undergoes fragmentation and conformational alterations, and these, as well as thiol oxidation, appear to be caused by hydroxyl radicals. Glycofluorophore formation is dependent upon ketoaldehyde formation. It is suggested that glucose autoxidation contributes to oxidative stress in pathophysiology associated with diabetes and aging via this newly described process of "autoxidative glycosylation".
The following report from Oct 30, 1981, shows the effects of glycation on cholesterol, LDL particles particularly and how it leads to atherosclerosis ;

- ### *Nonenzymatic glycosylation of low-density lipoproteins in vitro. Effects on cell-interactive properties*

Atherosclerosis occurs at an accelerated rate in patients with diabetes mellitus. Since some proteins undergo nonenzymatic glycosylation in diabetic patients and because certain chemical modifications of low-density

lipoproteins produced alterations in their interactions with certain cultured cells, a fact that may be relevant to atherogenesis, we investigated the effect of in vitro glycosylation on cell-related properties of low-density lipoproteins. Glycosylation was carried out by incubating LDL (1-10 mg LDL-protein/ml) with glucose (0-100 mM) in 0.5 M phosphate buffer, pH 8.0, at 37 degrees C. The amount of glucose incorporated into LDL after 1-2 wk of incubation was estimated to be in the range of 1-10 mol/mol LDL-protein. Amino acid analysis of glycosylated LDL showed that glucose was covalently bound to lysine residues. In studies with cultured human fibroblasts, glycosylated LDL was internalized and degraded significantly less than control LDL, in proportion to the estimated degree of glycosylation (12% of control for the most extensively glycosylated LDL). Glycosylation of LDL also impaired significantly its ability to stimulate cholesteryl ester synthesis in cultured fibroblasts. Glycosylated LDL did not stimulate cholesteryl ester synthesis in rat peritoneal macrophages. If glycosylation of LDL occurs in diabetic patients, some pathophysiologic consequences related to the increased incidence of atherosclerosis in these patients may result.
Study Link

In 1981 this was discovered, yet it's been 35 years since then and yet few people are aware of this. My question is, why? Maybe I should ask the sugar industry.

The following study shows the how the adhesive qualities of glucose creates fibrinogen, which becomes a target for glycation;

- **Polymerisation and crosslinking of fibrin monomers in diabetes mellitus**

Polymerisation and crosslinking of fibrin monomers were studied in 35 healthy volunteers and in 42 poorly controlled diabetic patients. Polymerisation did not show any difference between control subjects (n = 10) and diabetic patients (n = 11) (p greater than 0.1), although fibrinogen was 35% more glycated in the diabetic patients (p less than 0.001). Alpha chain crosslinking in the diabetic patients, however, was impaired as is shown from an increase in intermediate alpha polymers with a concomitant decrease in alpha monomer disappearance. A significant positive correlation was found between the degree of glycation of fibrinogen and the defective alpha chain polymerization (r = 0.86, p less than 0.005). These results were consistent with the results of thrombin and reptilase experiments. The reaction rate with reptilase did not show any difference between the two groups (p greater than 0.1), whereas the reaction rate with thrombin was significantly slower in the diabetic group compared to the control subjects (p less than 0.001). Purified fibrin clots obtained from the diabetic patients were more susceptible to plasmin than clots obtained from control subjects. It is concluded that in poorly controlled diabetic patients polymerization of fibrin monomers is normal, but crosslinking of the alpha chains is impaired, leading to a higher susceptibility of the clots to plasmin degradation.

From Wikipedia on Fibrinogen;

Fibrinogen (factor I) is a glycoprotein in vertebrates that helps in the formation of blood clots. It consists of a linear array of three nodules held together by a very thin thread which is estimated to have a diameter between 8 and 15 Angstrom (Å). The two end nodules are alike but the center one is slightly smaller. Measurements of shadow lengths indicate that nodule diameters are in the range 50 to 70 Å. The length of the dried molecule is 475 ± 25 Å.[2]

- ***Effect of low-density lipoprotein on the immunological determination glycation of apolipoprotein B***

Non-enzymatic glycation of low-density lipoprotein (LDL) may contribute to the premature atherogenesis of patients with diabetes mellitus. To assess whether glycation of apolipoprotein B, the predominant protein of LDL, interferes with the ability to immunologically quantify this protein, we prepared and purified glycated LDL by incubating normal plasma samples with high concentrations of glucose. Although both the plasma and the LDL specimens incubated with glucose contained significantly more glycated protein than control specimens, the quantitative interaction of an apolipoprotein B-specific antibody with glycated vs nonglycated LDL was not significantly different. We conclude that apolipoprotein B can be accurately quantified immunologically despite the presence of clinically excessive degrees of LDL glycation.
Study Link

I included the following study from November 1989 because of its explanation of how glycation is responsible for inflammation;

- ***Changes in concanavalin A-reactive proteins in inflammatory disorders***

Quantitative changes of concanavalin A (Con A)-reactive proteins in serum samples obtained from rats with induced inflammation and from patients with inflammatory and autoimmune diseases were examined by use of lectin blots. Treatment of rats with a single dose of fermented yeast to induce inflammation caused an extensive increase in Con A-reactivity. These changes were time-dependent and were similar in both sexes of the animals. When we examined serum samples obtained from patients with various inflammatory disorders for their Con A-reactive proteins as compared with normal donors, we noted that the Con A-reactivity increased in patients with rheumatoid arthritis and systemic lupus erythematosus. Among all the glycoproteins examined by lectin blots with use of Con A, a set of five proteins was selected for detailed analysis by densitometric scanning. These included alpha 2-macroglobulin, P-150, P-95, P-40, and P-35, of Mr 180,000, 150,000, 95,000, 40,000, and 35,000, respectively, by sodium dodecyl sulfate-polyacrylamide gel electrophoresis under reducing conditions. Densitometric scanning analysis of the lectin blots revealed that the Con A-reactivity of these proteins increased during inflammation. Because alpha 2-

macroglobulin is not an acute-phase protein in humans, an increase in Con A staining of this protein suggested that altered glycation is associated with autoimmune diseases. Thus, the study of changes in Con A-reactive proteins in human sera may facilitate our understanding of the etiology and pathophysiology of autoimmune diseases.   Study Link

- **Clinical Value of High Mobility Group Box 1 and the Receptor for Advanced Glycation End-products in Head and Neck Cancer: A Systematic Review**

"Abstract Introduction   High mobility group box 1 is a versatile protein involved in gene transcription, extracellular signaling, and response to inflammation. Extracellularly, high mobility group box 1 binds to several receptors, notably the receptor for advanced glycation end-products. Expression of high mobility group box 1 and the receptor for advanced glycation end-products has been described in many cancers. Objectives   To systematically review the available literature using PubMed and Web of Science to evaluate the clinical value of high mobility group box 1 and the receptor for advanced glycation end-products in head and neck squamous cell carcinomas. Data Synthesis   A total of eleven studies were included in this review. High mobility group box 1 overexpression is associated with poor prognosis and many clinical and pathological characteristics of head and neck squamous cell carcinomas patients. Additionally, the receptor for advanced glycation end-products demonstrates potential value as a clinical indicator of tumor angiogenesis and advanced staging. In diagnosis, high mobility group box 1 demonstrates low sensitivity. Conclusion   High mobility group box 1 and the receptor for advanced glycation end-products are associated with clinical and pathological characteristics of head and neck squamous cell carcinomas. Further investigation of the prognostic and diagnostic value of these molecules is warranted."

- **[Glycosylated lipoprotein]**

"Diabetes is frequently associated with cardiovascular diseases (coronary heart disease, cerebrovascular disease, peripheral vascular disease), and several risk factors have been proposed. Recent studies have strengthened the importance of chronic hyperglycemia because this modifies a variety of circulating substances including lipoproteins, and the glycosylated ones can be involved in the process of accelerating atherosclerosis. In this review, previous studies indicating the significance of glycosylated lipoproteins in the progression of atherosclerosis were overviewed. We also discussed AGE (advanced glycation end products) which may play an important role of atherogenesis in diabetes."The most recent study, submitted in October 2016 reveals some of the known damage that glycation is responsible for;

- **The relationship between plasma glycation with membrane modification, oxidative stress and expression of glucose transporter-1 in type 2 diabetes patients with vascular complications.**

BACKGROUND OF STUDY:
Enhanced protein glycation in diabetes causes irreversible cellular damage through membrane modifications. Erythrocytes are persistently exposed to plasma glycated proteins; however, little is known about its consequences on the membrane. The aim of this study was to examine the relationship between plasma protein glycation with erythrocyte membrane modifications in type 2 diabetes patients with and without vascular complications.
METHOD:
We recruited 60 healthy controls, 85 type 2 diabetic mellitus (DM) and 75 type 2 diabetic patients with complications (DMC). Levels of plasma glycation adduct with antioxidants (fructosamine, protein carbonyl, β-amyloids, thiol groups, total antioxidant status), erythrocyte membrane modifications (protein carbonyls, β-amyloids, free amino groups, erythrocyte fragility), antioxidant profile (GSH, catalase, lipid peroxidation) and Glut-1 expression were quantified.
RESULT:
Compared with controls, DM and DMC patients had significantly higher level of glycation adducts, erythrocyte fragility, lipid peroxidation and Glut-1 expression whereas declined levels of plasma and cellular antioxidants. Correlation studies revealed the positive association of membrane modifications with erythrocyte sedimentation rate, fragility, peroxidation whereas the negative association with free amino groups, glutathione, and catalase.
CONCLUSION:
Our data suggest that plasma glycation is associated with oxidative stress, Glut-1 expression and erythrocyte fragility in DM patients. This may further contribute to the progression of vascular complications.

More evidence of the role glucose plays in brain degradation;

- **Glycation potentiates neurodegeneration in models of Huntington's disease.**

Protein glycation is an age-dependent posttranslational modification associated with several neurodegenerative disorders, including Alzheimer's and Parkinson's diseases. By modifying amino-groups, glycation interferes with the folding of proteins, increasing their aggregation potential. Here, we studied the effect of pharmacological and genetic manipulation of glycation on huntingtin (HTT), the causative protein in Huntington's disease (HD). We observed that glycation increased the aggregation of mutant HTT exon 1 fragments associated with HD (HTT72Q and HTT103Q) in yeast and mammalian cell models. We found that glycation impairs HTT clearance thereby promoting its intracellular accumulation and aggregation.

Interestingly, under these conditions autophagy increased and the levels of mutant HTT released to the culture medium decreased. Furthermore, increased glycation enhanced HTT toxicity in human cells and neurodegeneration in fruit flies, impairing eclosion and decreasing lifespan. Overall, our study provides evidence that glycation modulates HTT exon-1 aggregation and toxicity, and suggests it may constitute a novel target for therapeutic intervention in HD.

Brain development hinges on the cholesterol as well, as cholesterol is your brain's neuronal-connectors. It couldn't operate without it. This report illustrates the importance of cholesterol in the brain;

- ***Cholesterol in brain disease: sometimes determinant and frequently implicated***
Cholesterol is essential for neuronal physiology, both during development and in the adult life: as a major component of cell membranes and precursor of steroid hormones, it contributes to the regulation of ion permeability, cell shape, cell-cell interaction, and transmembrane signaling. Consistently, hereditary diseases with mutations in cholesterol-related genes result in impaired brain function during early life. In addition, defects in brain cholesterol metabolism may contribute to neurological syndromes, such as Alzheimer's disease (AD), Huntington's disease (HD), and Parkinson's disease (PD), and even to the cognitive deficits typical of the old age. In these cases, brain cholesterol defects may be secondary to disease-causing elements and contribute to the functional deficits by altering synaptic functions. In the first part of this review, we will describe hereditary and non-hereditary causes of cholesterol dyshomeostasis and the relationship to brain diseases. In the second part, we will focus on the mechanisms by which perturbation of cholesterol metabolism can affect synaptic function. In summary, it is clear that a direct disturbance of cholesterol metabolism, for example, by defects in cholesterol synthesizing enzymes or transporters, impairs brain development and function. In addition, changes in cholesterol metabolism in the adult and during aging, and in several age-related neurodegenerative diseases, can directly impact on brain function.
Another report disputes the dangers of cholesterol in this report dated Feb 18, 2012;

Is the use of cholesterol in mortality risk algorithms in clinical guidelines valid? Ten years prospective data from the Norwegian HUNT 2 study
Many clinical guidelines for cardiovascular disease (CVD) prevention contain risk estimation charts/calculators. These have shown a tendency to overestimate risk, which indicates that there might be theoretical flaws in the algorithms. Total cholesterol is a frequently used variable in the risk estimates. Some studies indicate that the predictive properties of cholesterol might not be as straightforward as widely assumed. Our aim was to document the strength and validity of total cholesterol as a risk factor for

mortality in a well-defined, general Norwegian population without known CVD at baseline.
Conclusions
Based on epidemiological analysis of updated and comprehensive population data, we found that the underlying assumptions regarding cholesterol in clinical guidelines for CVD prevention might be flawed: cholesterol emerged as an overestimated risk factor in our study, indicating that guideline information might be misleading, particularly for women with 'moderately elevated' cholesterol levels in the range of 5–7 mmol L−1. Our findings are in good accord with some previous studies. A potential explanation of the lack of accord between clinical guidelines and recent population data, including ours, is time trend changes for CVD/IHD and underlying causal (risk) factors.
Conclusion
Our study provides an updated epidemiological indication of possible errors in the CVD risk algorithms of many clinical guidelines. If our findings are generalizable, clinical and public health recommendations regarding the 'dangers' of cholesterol should be revised. This is especially true for women, for whom moderately elevated cholesterol (by current standards) may prove to be not only harmless but even beneficial.

The previous report disputes the often fatal assumption that high cholesterol is hazardous to your health. They're recommending a change is advice offered.

- ***Extracellular HMGB1 promotes differentiation of nurse-like cells in chronic lymphocytic leukemia***

"Chronic lymphocytic leukemia (CLL) is a disease of an accumulation of mature B cells that are highly dependent on the microenvironment for maintenance and expansion. However, little is known regarding the mechanisms whereby CLL cells create their favorable microenvironment for survival. High-mobility group protein B-1 (HMGB1) is a highly conserved nuclear protein that can be actively secreted by innate immune cells and passively released by injured or dying cells. We found significantly increased HMGB1 levels in the plasma of CLL patients compared with healthy controls, and HMGB1 concentration is associated with absolute lymphocyte count. We, therefore, sought to determine potential roles of HMGB1 in modulating the CLL microenvironment. CLL cells passively released HMGB1, and the timing and concentrations of HMGB1 in the medium were associated with differentiation of nurse-like cells (NLCs). Higher CD68 expression in CLL lymph nodes, one of the markers for NLCs, was associated with shorter overall survival of CLL patients. HMGB1-mediated NLC differentiation involved internalization of both receptors for advanced glycation end products (RAGE) and Toll-like receptor-9 (TLR9). Differentiation of NLCs can be prevented by blocking the HMGB1-RAGE-TLR9 pathway. In conclusion,

this study demonstrates for the first time that CLL cells might modulate their microenvironment by releasing HMGB1."   Free PMC Article
J Clin Invest. *1984 Nov;74(5):1742-9.*

After searching these last few disorders I got a yen to search any disorder & glycation, and glycation turned up in everything except halitosis. The following report shows its involvement in stomach ulcers. I originally searched just ulcers and got back 30 studies showing involvement. The first few studies in the list were reports on foot ulcers, so I search stomach ulcers and found 3 studies, the following report was the first;

- **High-mobility group box 1 inhibits gastric_ulcer_healing through Toll-like receptor 4 and receptor for advanced_glycation_end products**

High-mobility group box 1 (HMGB1) was initially discovered as a nuclear protein that interacts with DNA as a chromatin-associated non-histone protein to stabilize nucleosomes and to regulate the transcription of many genes in the nucleus. Once leaked or actively secreted into the extracellular environment, HMGB1 activates inflammatory pathways by stimulating multiple receptors, including Toll-like receptor (TLR) 2, TLR4, and receptor for advanced glycation end products (RAGE), leading to tissue injury. Although HMGB1's ability to induce inflammation has been well documented, no studies have examined the role of HMGB1 in wound healing in the gastrointestinal field. The aim of this study was to evaluate the role of HMGB1 and its receptors in the healing of gastric ulcers. We also investigated which receptor among TLR2, TLR4, or RAGE mediates HMGB1's effects on ulcer healing. Gastric ulcers were induced by serosal application of acetic acid in mice, and gastric tissues were processed for further evaluation. The induction of ulcer increased the immunohistochemical staining of cytoplasmic HMGB1 and elevated serum HMGB1 levels. Ulcer size, myeloperoxidase (MPO) activity, and the expression of tumor necrosis factor α (TNFα) mRNA peaked on day 4. Intraperitoneal administration of HMGB1 delayed ulcer healing and elevated MPO activity and TNFα expression. In contrast, administration of anti-HMGB1 antibody promoted ulcer healing and reduced MPO activity and TNFα expression. TLR4 and RAGE deficiency enhanced ulcer healing and reduced the level of TNFα, whereas ulcer healing in TLR2 knockout (KO) mice was similar to that in wild-type mice. In TLR4 KO and RAGE KO mice, exogenous HMGB1 did not affect ulcer healing and TNFα expression. Thus, we showed that HMGB1 is a complicating factor in the gastric ulcer healing process, which acts through TLR4 and RAGE to induce excessive inflammatory responses.   Free PMC Article

- **Nonenzymatic glycation of human lens crystallin, Effect of aging and diabetes mellitus**

Garlick RL, Mazer JS, Chylack LT Jr, Tung WH, Bunn HF.

This study looked at the effects of glycation on your eyes and cataracts it's responsible for. Yes, glycation and a glucose diet will buy you cataracts. My mother had two of them. A good friend who loved to eat her bread had cataracts in both of her eyes as well. What's interesting, this person was always complaining of headaches and stomach aches. Both of those manifestations are from an ECC diet. Again, here is more evidence of the glycative and addictive effects of a grain diet. In all, there were 3,629 studies on the effects of glucose glycating proteins, hemoglobin, and cholesterol dating back to March 1984. Incidentally, that was one month after I was released from the hospital after spending a month in a coma and suffering two strokes while comatose. I could have never come back this far without Dr. Perlmutter's help. Again, I have to thank you, Dr. Perlmutter.

They've had some of this evidence for over 30 years, why hasn't the public been told about glycation or the AGEs they create? It's those AGEs that are at the root of all modern diseases. If this was uncovered starting 30+ years ago, why have we just found out about it from the bestselling books from two doctors? Is someone trying to hide something? My guess is yes. This is Monsanto's path to power and freedom. They've politically engineered their freedom to wreak whatever havoc they can on your health by masturbating your taste buds with their glucose laden products, to grant them power by buying into their pharmaceutical cycle in the very near future. By near, I mean, it only takes a couple days before you're indebted. (That means addicted.) If you want true power and freedom, you can have it in two weeks to two months. That's how long it takes to break the addiction.

Each and every one of these 11,000+ studies has been vetted and examined by the NIH and PubMed for whom I thank immensely. It's clear that this *ruse/problem/pandemic* is not going to go away unless the consumer does something about it, them. The only way out of this dilemma leaves you with very limited options,

You have two choices;

1. Continue to masturbate your taste buds and collect these diseases and disorders in return.
2. Cut out as much as possible the starchy carbohydrates, (grains) and live free from dependence.

You need to realize that the comfort in comfort food, brings massive discomfort in the future, and the process starts immediately, with a process called glycation. This is the real poisoning of America and we can correct it. It lies within our power. Each and every one of us can correct this. I offer a cure, not a therapy or treatment, My cure simply involves removal of all glycating substances from the diet to eliminate this problem of glycation so that it never affects the body The glycating substances = carbs, sugar, glucose, fructose.

The above reports on the effects of glycation appeared in some cases, over 30 years ago in PubMed. Many of these reports were submitted just last year, as those are the first ones I come across. I've only shown you a few of the reports out of 11,850 studies to date detailing the damaging effects of Excessive Carbohydrate Consumption, the primary cause of glycation, why doesn't the FDA or the USDA say anything about that? The 42nd study, submitted in November 1989 shows how it causes inflammation, and with inflammation a factor in so many diseases, it truly is a wonder that the FDA and USDA never even issued anything so simple as a warning. The FDA'S INVOLVEMENT in this issue is mostly explained by their influence from the one industry, where they get most of their execs from, Monsanto.

From every form of cancer to Alzheimer's disease to heart disease and cardiovascular disease to arthritis to hypertension to high cholesterol these food sources (sugar and grains) are responsible for each and every one of these disorders. These studies are proof of exactly what sugar does to the body. To cure the glycation factor in these diseases, the best way is to eliminate it as much as possible. To do that you must eliminate its source and to eliminate the source, you have to eliminate the grains and sugar. Thank you, Dr. Davis and Dr. Perlmutter, for bringing this to my attention.

In all, there were 3,629 studies in the FDA's database on the effects of glucose glycating proteins, hemoglobin, and cholesterol dating back to march, 1984. Incidentally, that was one month after I was released from the hospital after spending a month in a coma and suffering two strokes while comatose. I could have never come back this far without Dr. Perlmutter's help. Again, I have to thank you, Dr. Perlmutter. The above, reports on the effects of glycation, appeared, in some cases over 30 years ago in PubMed or PMC. With 11,667 studies to date in PubMed, detailing the damaging effects of Excessive Carbohydrate Consumption, the primary cause of glycation, why doesn't the FDA say anything? There are roughly 6,000 more studies in PMC. The last study, submitted in November 1989 shows how it causes inflammation and with inflammation a factor in so many diseases, it truly is a wonder that the FDA never even issued anything as simple as a warning. The **FDA's involvement** in this issue is largely explained by the influence they receive from the one industry where they get a good portion of their execs from, Monsanto.

While having the evidence for over 30 years, why hasn't the public been told about glycation or the AGEs they create? It's those AGEs that are at the root of all modern diseases. If this was uncovered 30+ years ago, why have we just found out about it from the bestselling books from two doctors? Why did it take these two doctors to inform us of what's been going on? Why wasn't it the FDA or the USDA? Isn't that their job?

It would have been nice if someone could have warned me about this 20 or 30 years ago but the USDA and FDA had different ideas. For that, I thank Monsanto. Don't allow them to be in your driver's seat. As long as you remain on your carbohydrate diet, they're in the driver's seat for your health. Give up the carbs and put yourself back in the driver's seat. You are the only one who can change yourself. Enable yourself to do so.

Documentaries worth watching;

1. Food, Inc

2. Food Matters

3. Food Beware (French)

4. Genetically Modified Foods

5. David vs Monsanto

6. Of the Land

7. Hungry for Change

8. That Sugar Film

9. Fathead

10. Love Paleo

11. Heal Yourself

12. Fresh

13. Overfed and Undernourished

14. My Big Fat Body

15. Facing the Fat

16. Fat

17. Who Wants to Live Forever

Chapter 6

Why I Stay In Ketosis

Ketosis refers to acids in the body that are derived and used while in a state of low glucose in the blood. Because my body has been in a state of ketosis for the last 3 years, I feel qualified to speak about this lifestyle. I call it a lifestyle because it really is. It's a lifestyle completely different from the lifestyle of a carboholic. It's a lifestyle that's not subject to the hunger cycle.

Carboholics require food every other hour or so, it's the law of carb consumption, appetite follows glucose levels in the blood. It's that simple, blood sugar levels rise and satiety sets in, releasing hormones controlling feel-good emotions influencing behavior, sometimes unrecognizable behavior. But, that usually happens when the blood sugars fall again after a couple hours releasing hormones of hunger, need and want. These hormones are completely different than the satiety hormones and have many different effects on the body. I submit that it's this change in the hormonal influence that drives most behavior on the planet.

In my estimation, this change in our hormones is what drives a major portion of our abhorrent behavior today. This is what drives terrorism, by driving anger by driving the hunger cycle. It's my contention that if this hunger cycle can be controlled, you can control all anger and terrorism.

In this chapter, I'm going to explain the advantages of not being controlled by the hunger cycle because I believe that it's this hunger cycle that lies behind all despicable behavior. Breaking this hunger cycle puts you back in control of your own emotions and in doing so, puts you back in control of your own behavior.

According to PubMed, on the subject of ketosis;

"Hunger and satiety are two important mechanisms involved in body weight regulation. Even though humans can regulate food intake by will, there are systems within the central nervous system (CNS) that regulate food intake and energy expenditure. This complex network, whose control center is spread over different brain areas, receives information from adipose tissue, the gastrointestinal tract (GIT), and from blood and peripheral sensory receptors. The actions of the brain's hunger/satiety centers are influenced by nutrients, hormones and other signaling molecules. Ketone bodies are the major source of energy in the periods of fasting and/or carbohydrate shortage and might play a role in food intake control."

They go on to say; *"Glucose also exerts a hormonal-like action on neurons; electrophysiological recordings demonstrated, for example, that hypoglycemia activates growth hormone-releasing hormone (GHRH) neurons, suggesting a mechanistic link between low blood glucose levels and growth hormone release (Stanley et al., 2013)."*

This is where carboholics cannot have the advantages that being in a state of nutritional ketosis has. Those who chose to live in a state of ketosis) aren't controlled by their hormones, so they don't have to follow any hunger cycle. They're in full control of their hormones. With hormones being the primary driver of appetite (Leptin & Ghrelin), they influence your appetite more than anything and are able to alter your ability to discern whether you need to eat or not. It's called leptin resistance and we'll get deeper into that later.

This also means that these hormones are in control of your emotions, because of that. I know that it doesn't sound like it's that big of a deal, but it's more important than you ever could imagine. As explained in *Why the addiction is so hard to break*, it has to do with how your hormones control your actions without you realizing it.

First, let's look at the state of ketosis, as explained in Wikipedia;

"Ketosis /kɪˈtoʊsɪs/ IS A METABOLIC STATE IN WHICH MOST OF THE BODY'S ENERGY SUPPLY COMES FROM ketone bodies IN THE BLOOD, IN CONTRAST TO A STATE OF glycolysis IN WHICH blood glucose PROVIDES MOST OF THE ENERGY. KETOSIS IS SIMILAR TO A CONDITION CALLED KETOACIDOSIS, IN THAT BOTH CAUSE A SIDE EFFECT KNOWN TO LAYPEOPLE AS acetone breath. LONGER-TERM KETOSIS MAY RESULT FROM fasting OR STAYING ON A LOW-CARBOHYDRATE DIET AND DELIBERATELY INDUCED KETOSIS SERVES AS A MEDICAL INTERVENTION FOR VARIOUS CONDITIONS, SUCH AS INTRACTABLE EPILEPSY, AND THE VARIOUS TYPES OF DIABETES. IN GLYCOLYSIS, HIGHER LEVELS OF INSULIN PROMOTE STORAGE OF BODY FAT AND BLOCK RELEASE OF FAT FROM ADIPOSE TISSUES, WHILE IN KETOSIS, FAT RESERVES ARE READILY RELEASED AND CONSUMED. FOR THIS REASON, KETOSIS IS SOMETIMES REFERRED TO AS THE BODY'S "FAT BURNING" MODE."

This biggest problem with a state of ketosis is that it is often confused with ketoacidosis, which has nothing to do with being in a state of nutritional ketosis. Ketoacidosis is a state of extreme ketosis that can only happen to type 1 diabetics because their pancreas is incapable of secreting enough insulin to handle even a small amount of glucose in the system. Because of this the liver of type 1 diabetics secretes more ketones than what the body needs to operate. Again Wikipedia says;

The worst mistake one can make about ketosis is to confuse it with Ketosis-Onset Diabetes or Ketosis-Prone Diabetes. These are conditions of extreme diabetes in which the body can't supply enough insulin for the amount of glucose in the body. It's explained in this report from Apr 23, 2013;

Ketosis-Onset Diabetes and Ketosis-Prone Diabetes: Same or Not?
Ketosis-prone diabetes (KPD) is defined as a widespread, emerging, heterogeneous syndrome characterized by patients who present with DKA or unprovoked ketosis but do not necessarily have the typical phenotype of autoimmune type 1 diabetes
While ketosis-onset diabetes patients present with ketosis or ketoacidosis without known diabetes, some investigators defined ketosis-onset diabetes as diabetes with the presence of diabetic ketosis and in the absence of glutamic acid decarboxylase (GAD) and tyrosin phosphatase (IA-2) autoantibodies.

Both of those conditions are manifestations of Diabetic Ketoacidosis (DKA). These conditions have little if anything to do with nutritional ketosis.

Although I appreciate nutritional ketosis as being a "fat burning mode", it's the other benefits that I appreciate more. I get to live with benefits like less pain, no headaches, no stomach aches, far more energy than what I've ever had, and the ability to get far more work done as I don't have to stop all the time, to eat. My efficiency in the last 6 – 12 months has been nothing short of phenomenal and although I do eat at my desk, I'm usually at my desk 16-18 hours out of the day, except on therapy days. I take 3 hours, 3 days a week for therapy. My therapy is exercise. My brain needs it, but my body benefits.

BY INSULIN DEFICIENCY, HYPERGLYCEMIA, AND DEHYDRATION. PARTICULARLY IN TYPE 1 DIABETICS THE LACK OF INSULIN IN THE BLOODSTREAM PREVENTS GLUCOSE ABSORPTION, THEREBY INHIBITING THE PRODUCTION OF OXALOACETATE (A CRUCIAL PRECURSOR TO THE B-OXIDATION OF FATTY ACIDS) THROUGH REDUCED LEVELS OF PYRUVATE (A BYPRODUCT OF GLYCOLYSIS), AND CAN CAUSE UNCHECKED KETONE BODY PRODUCTION (THROUGH FATTY ACID METABOLISM) POTENTIALLY LEADING TO DANGEROUS GLUCOSE AND KETONE LEVELS IN THE BLOOD. HYPERGLYCEMIA RESULTS IN GLUCOSE OVERLOADING THE KIDNEYS AND SPILLING INTO THE URINE (TRANSPORT MAXIMUM FOR GLUCOSE IS EXCEEDED). DEHYDRATION RESULTS, FOLLOWING THE OSMOTIC MOVEMENT OF WATER INTO URINE. (OSMOTIC DIURESIS), EXACERBATES THE ACIDOSIS."

I bring this up to make the point that nutritional ketosis is not ketoacidosis. It's far from it. According to Wikipedia again, *"NORMAL serum reference ranges FOR KETONE BODIES ARE 0.5–3.0 MG/DL, EQUIVALENT TO 0.05–0.29 MMOL/L."*

In ketosis, the levels range from 3 – 6 mg/dL. Ketoacidosis requires a level of 15 – 25 mg/dL, more than three times the levels needed for ketosis, making it virtually impossible for anyone to go into ketoacidosis if you're not a type 1 diabetic. Actually, ketoacidosis happens when the body is overloaded with carbs and can't produce enough insulin to convert the sugar and turns to ketones in a panic. This condition requires an overload of sugar to produce the reaction. That is the last thing a diabetic wants to do. Nutritional ketosis has been instrumental in treating type2 diabetes.

Remaining in a state of ketosis and not depending on sugar, on the other hand, has allowed my body to regain that which was lost 32 years ago in a car accident that left me severely disabled because of a severe closed head injury, (It was the two strokes that were the most devastating.)

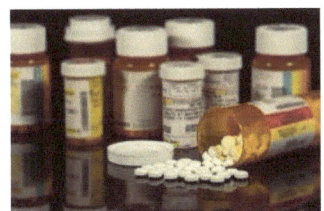

DRUGS THAT I WON'T NEED ANYMORE

Probably the first and foremost reason I choose to remain on this diet is explained by my lack of need for any of these diabetes medications. I just can't afford them or the side effects that they carry with them;

insulin, exenatide, liraglutide, pramlintide, Biguanides, metformin
Phenformin- Phenformin (DBI) WAS USED FROM THE 1960S THROUGH 1980S BUT WAS WITHDRAWN DUE TO TO LACTIC ACIDOSIS RISK.
Buformin - ALSO WAS WITHDRAWN DUE TO LACTIC ACIDOSIS RISK.
Thiazolidinediones;
Rosiglitazone - (AVANDIA): THE European Medicines Agency RECOMMENDED IN SEPTEMBER 2010 THAT IT BE SUSPENDED FROM THE EU MARKET DUE TO ELEVATED CARDIOVASCULAR RISKS.
Pioglitazone
Troglitazone - (REZULIN): USED IN 1990S, WITHDRAWN DUE TO hepatitis AND LIVER DAMAGE RISK
PEPTIDE ANALOGS; Secretagogues;
FIRST-GENERATION AGENTS; tolbutamide, acetohexamide, tolazamide, chlorpropamide
SECOND-GENERATION AGENTS; glipizide, glyburide or glibenclamide, glimepiride, gliclazide, gliquidone, Meglitinides, repaglinide, nateglinide, Alpha-glucosidase inhibitors, miglitol, acarbose, voglibose.
INJECTABLE AMYLIN ANALOGUES
Amylin, pramlintide, SGLT-2 inhibitors
COMMON GENERIC NAMES FOR MANY OF THESE MEDICINES ARE FROM WIKIPEDIA; MANY ANTI-DIABETES DRUGS ARE AVAILABLE AS GENERICS. THESE INCLUDE:[35]
Sulfonylureas- GLIMEPIRIDE, GLIPIZIDE, GLYBURIDE
Biguanides- METFORMIN
Thiazolidinediones(TZD) - PIOGLITAZONE, ACTOS GENERIC
Alpha-glucosidase inhibitors- ACARBOSE
Meglitinides- NATEGLINIDE
Combination of sulfonylureas plus metformin - known by generic names of the two drugs

The above medications are used for diabetes alone. This small list is quite possibly the smallest list that one will need to choose from with a continued diet of carbohydrates. Larger lists exist for heart disease, cancer, high blood pressure, high cholesterol, arthritis, and dementia. That only covers the prescription medication. For OCD medication, you have to consider NSAIDs, the most used pain relievers all carrying more side effects to create more need for further medication. And don't forget Tylenol. How many problems does that drug have with liver toxicity? It's been responsible for a few deaths.

Then we have to look at the Antacids and all the stomach medicine that's on the shelf. There are plenty of them and I can honestly tell you right now that

90% of these medications are not necessary unless you're on a carbohydrate diet. I haven't used any of these medications in 3 years since I gave up the bread and carbs. I used to have two or three volumes of drug catalogs full of pharmaceuticals that are needed to treat all of the diseases that are caused by the consumption of grains, from diabetes to dementia to heart disease and cancer. My first post lists all of those.

I refuse to take any of these drugs anymore because all of them carry side effects, some major, some minor. Whether the side effects are major or minor, I don't want to experience any of them. I've had my fill of side effects, especially the ones that make my health worse, which is where most of these side effects should be classified. After living for twenty years need to take massive amounts of opioids for my chronic severe pain, diuretics for my high blood pressure, anti-depressants for the pain, and living with the side effects of not only the opioids but every other drug they had me on, all twelve of them. I'm fed up with it. I'm not going to take it anymore. And I was only up to twelve medications. I have a friend who's on this diet, who's lowered his needs to thirteen daily medications from twenty-three. How many meds do you take every day?

I prefer the theory that if the meds aren't needed in the first place, my health is going to be that much better. That is why I removed everything from my diet that I could, that is responsible for these horrendous diseases, requiring the need for these medications. The one thread I found that ties 90% of all cancers (even lung cancer), 90% of all heart diseases, and 99.9 % of all dementia, all arthritis, all headaches, and almost all stomach aches together is one substance that can be removed from the diet without any severe side effects. I shouldn't need to tell you what that substance is by now. You should know. You eat it every day. You live with the effects of addiction. Pain always comes with addiction.

You eat it every morning, either in your coffee as creamer, in the toast you have, or the cereal you consume. You have it every lunch with your sandwich or burrito and with every dinner with your rolls. I have known several families that would just put a plate of bread on the table every evening. This is the display of addiction, a full out need to satisfy the taste buds by dumping more and more sugar in the body, usually in the form of starchy carbs.

The sad part of this whole argument is that I've only covered drugs for diabetes so far. I haven't even touched on drugs for heart disease, cancer, arthritis, high blood pressure, high cholesterol (probably the most dangerous), chronic pain, hyperlipidemia, obesity, etc, etc. How many side effects do think all these drugs can cause? How many more avenues can this create to develop new drugs to spring upon a mindless public clamoring for the newest drug of relief for their pain?

All of this consumption of the grain industry's products is what's driving the pharmaceutical industry today, tomorrow, next year, and will continue to drive it for the next 500 years and beyond. If we don't put an end to this now, our society is doomed to suffer the consequences of their carbohydrate addiction, a diet they're not responsible for. The greed of the grain industry combined with the ambition of the pharmaceutical industry has made us all carboholic slaves to the desires these industries. Just like the alcoholic is a slave to the liquor industry, the carboholic's masters are the grain and pharmaceutical industries. For me, it's scary how much power we've given these industries, simply because we listen to their advertising. Those who take their message to heart, and are influenced by it, fall prey to that influence and become their slaves for life or until they quit consuming the grains. It's an addiction that differs little from that of alcoholism. (Fortunately, the withdrawal symptoms aren't as bad.)

Anyone who can't control their emotions entirely by themselves is a slave to their own emotions. All addicts who recognize their addiction knows this to be true. Every addict follows their emotions before following anything else. That's because it's only their emotions that will feed the addiction. Common sense won't. It's the hormones, though that control your emotions.

Every carboholic is a slave to their hormones and hence a slave to their emotions and therefore a slave to these industries. The emotions I'm speaking about here are hunger and satiety. You may not classify these emotions, but I submit that they actually are. Satiety is defined as the state of being satisfied. If that is not an emotion, as it expresses feelings of calmness and security, I don't know what is. Hunger, on the other hand, is defined as a strong desire. Is not that an emotion? These emotions are controlled by both leptin and Ghrelin, which in turn are controlled by the grain industry, more than anything else. I refuse to take part in this trap anymore.

With emotions being controlled by our hormonal balance like this, how could the influence of anything that modifies that balance, not has an effect on our behavior? It has to. When you combine the drive of an addiction (which is what we're talking about) with the advertisements promoting that addiction, how can it not have an effect on our health and ultimately our society? That is why I make the statement that this cycle has to change. If it doesn't cease, our health as a society will never get better.

Let's go back to addiction, though, for I'm sure you don't consider this an addiction. I understand few caught in an addiction can recognize that addiction when they're feeding it because the addiction has ways of hiding it. You can ask anyone who has to have at least one beer a day. They're not addicted to their beer, as far as they're concerned, yet they have to have it. And often they don't even drink more than just one. But they still have to have that one. That is what makes it an addiction. The body can and does live much better without beer, so it's not a substance the body requires to survive. Yet the beer drinker needs that daily beer to satisfy their addiction.

To go without, many times causes more problems because of the work your hormones are doing on your emotions and worse yet your actions by controlling how receptors work in your brain. That makes it a natural thing that you need to do, and not an addiction, to appease that desire to drink the beer. This is how addiction works and it happens to carboholics too. I know I am a carboholic. The desire for sweets is still with me. It's the last refuge of my addiction. It's something that I get to fight for the rest of my life.

When I think about this I get angry, for I never asked for this nor could I ever wish for it, or wish it upon anyone else. Yet, there is an industry that is committed to not only continuing this pattern, they're goal is to increase its scope. You can see this in all the advertising.

What do you think they're advertising promotes when they show you feel good commercials for their soft drinks, fruit drinks, cereals, bread, pasta, pastries, candy, etc, etc? They're using your emotions to control your behavior. That's because they can. They already control your hormones and it's your hormones that control your emotions. Is it any wonder that so many are addicted? This is the cycle of addiction that I avoid by being on my keto diet. I also avoid the cycle of hunger that everyone one carb diet has to deal with. This may be the best-unexpected benefit of a keto diet. No more cycles of pain and hunger. No more, do cycles of anger and contentment bother me nor do any cycles of fear, hate, and rage, thanks to my keto diet.

This industry has taken my right to chose simply by addicting me more, to a substance that has far deadlier consequences than it has ever had in the past. In my estimation, this is criminal behavior. It's criminal behavior being done on an industrial level. That is why I posted yesterday's post on our celebration of addiction. They do this because they know that we are addicted to our rate of consumption of their wares. They also know that with their lobbying power, they can get away with virtually anything. It's kind of the same situation as that of the military-industrial complex. They support congressmen and senators in every state and district, securing their interests, with this influence. There are very few districts or states that don't support farming, yet we allow this abuse to happen, for which we should be ashamed.

Because Monsanto is a corporation, the Supreme Court has determined that they deserve the same rights as an individual even though they don't have same moral values that most individuals have. Those who do criminal deeds we put in jail, but it's hard to put a corporation in jail for its criminal deeds.

We've made it legal for them to sell us their food contaminated with their glyphosate herbicides, regardless of how much cancer it causes. If this isn't criminal behavior, I don't know what is. That may be due to the fact that one of our Supreme Court Justices used to be an attorney for Monsanto in the late 70's. Clarence Thomas may go down in history as the Justice who did more to contribute to the ill health of America than any other Justice. I wonder how many deaths he's responsible for.

This is just a small iota of Monsanto's drive for profit. Justice Thomas wrote the decision that allowed Monsanto to patent something as simple as a seed. I wonder if his severance package left him with any stock options when he left Monsanto? This is what allows Monsanto to force farmers to grow their GMO seed, whether they want to or not. This is the evil of industrial farming, engineered Monsanto style, courtesy of Justice Thomas.

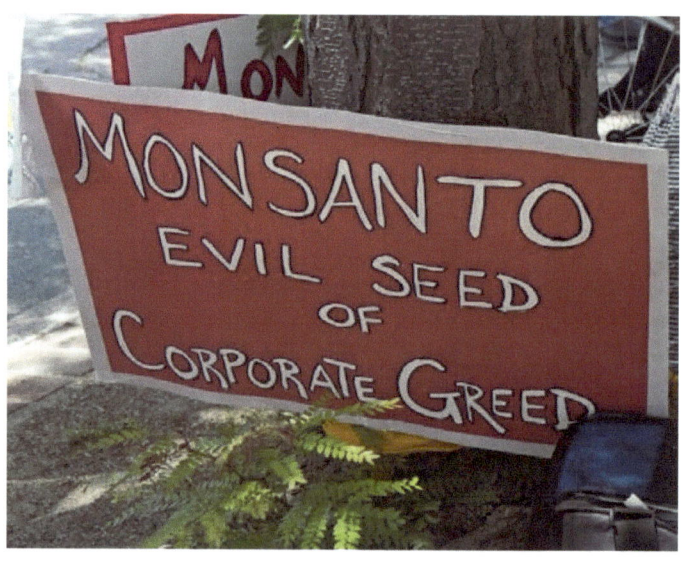

Chapter 7

The Grain Industry's Ruse to Feed You Disease

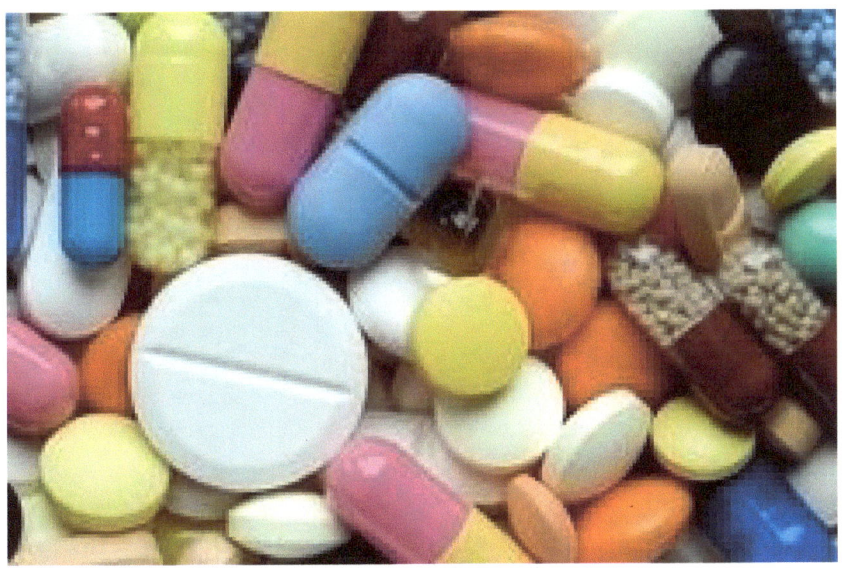

My father disposed of a 1 gallon Ziploc bag full of these drugs after my mother died - $421,324.83 worth.

This is a matter of your health being engineered without your knowledge or consent. The engineering, in this case, is not good. Actually, it's creating pain where none should exist. Our food supply industry may be the most important industry concerned when it comes to our health. As everyone knows, 'you are what you eat', so it's vital that what you eat won't make you sick. Unfortunately, for those who still masturbate their taste buds with their addiction to sugar, this couldn't be further from the truth. Our food supply has been hijacked by the same industry that treats you for the illness their food supplies. Granted the healthcare industry is vital to our health, but I submit that it wouldn't be as important as it is today if we paid more attention to what we eat.

Because I now watch what I eat, I can change the "we" to "you", meaning "you" have to watch what you eat. (All that means is that you still have an addiction to break, I don't, I broke mine three years ago.) Because of this addiction, you've doomed yourself unwittingly to a lifetime of medications. That is unless you're one of the .05% who shows no ill effects from glycation.

I have yet to meet one of them. If you eat at a restaurant or buy groceries at a grocery store, you're subject to this addiction. It's in their food everywhere you look. You actually look for it because you love to eat it. You love their advertising. What's not to love, it's full of attractive people selling you what appears to provide health, but in all reality provides nothing but the opposite, as it's responsible for most all pain, most all disease, all brain damage, all atherosclerosis, all diseases affiliated with inflammation, and this is just for starters.

Monsanto has politically engineered their dominance of your food supply and subsequent health by forcing as many farmers as they can to use Monsanto's seed companies' GMO seed to grow their crops. Monsanto has many seed companies. Their control over the seed industry was mirrored by their control over the pharmaceutical industry because they could use the seed companies to influence the profits of their drug companies. Monsanto owns 15 crop seed companies all selling GMO seed for their contracted farmers to grow. Five of these companies sell seed for wheat crops. That's the seed that grows the wheat that's ground into flour for your bread and crackers.

 Their contracted farmers have to grow Monsanto's GMO seed at risk of facing legal action if caught growing anything else. This is how Monsanto controls what goes on your table to eat. This is also how Monsanto forces you into purchasing the CELEBREX, made by Searle Pharmaceuticals. Searle had been part of Monsanto from 1985 – 2003 when it was sold to Pfizer along with the rest of Pharmacia. The Celebrex is what your doctor prescribes for your arthritis that's caused by the glycation set up from the grain diet you've been on all your life. After you get arthritis that you will inevitably get from eating their GMO grains, you'll be begging your doctor for that prescription for the Celebrex.

Then you'll get to deal with the side effects of the Celebrex that it inevitably presents to the body. That's the damage to your body from the drug side of their industry. The damage from the crop seed side includes crops that are not only GMO seed, they are laden with Roundup, the glyphosate herbicide that works by inhibiting enzymes from doing what they supposed to do by instructing cells how to operate. Even though Monsanto claims that these enzyme inhibitors affect only targeted enzymes, the rise in cancer alone, that the nation has seen since the mid to late 80's, has told a completely different story.

The rise in these disorders is directly caused by an increase in the glycation that occurs in the blood by the high glucose laden grains this company forces their farmers to grow. That means that the food going on your table is engineered to make you need the medications that the pharmaceutical companies sell. This makes me wonder if a hidden clause in their merger is forcing Monsanto to provide customers for their old pharmaceutical companies. I know you haven't considered the possibility, but I would suggest that you do, your health is at risk. (It's probably many clauses in many contracts involving stock options.) That's the only thing I can think of that could drive this behavior for the USDA and the FDA.

According to Wikipedia; *"IN DECEMBER, 1997 MONSANTO MERGED WITH PHARMACIA AND UPJOHN. THE AGRICULTURAL DIVISION BECAME A WHOLLY OWNED SUBSIDIARY OF THE "NEW" PHARMACIA; MONSANTO'S MEDICAL RESEARCH DIVISION, WHICH INCLUDED PRODUCTS SUCH AS CELEBREX."*

Searle and Pharmacia were the other sides of Monsanto's multinational chemical companies that includes Upjohn as well. Searle merged with Monsanto in 1985 two years after Monsanto started dabbling in GMO crops. In 1993 Searle filed for a patent for Celebrex, its widely used arthritis drug. I'll bet you didn't know that it is Monsanto's seed companies that force their contracted farmers to grow GMO seed designed to make you need their Celebrex. Is this what you thought you were buying when you bought those corn chips last time? Was this what you thought you were buying when you purchased those pretzels?

Whether or not it was, that's what you got. You also got all the rest of the damage that glycation does to the body, which includes atherosclerosis, cancer, and dementia as well. You're also subjecting yourself to the hunger cycle, probably the worst manifestation of a carb diet. The more carbs you eat, the hungrier you get. That's a cycle that can't be broken if you don't stop the fuel that feeds it. Stopping the fuel is the only way to stop the glycation. That means that it's the only way to stop the inflammation, which means it's the only way to stop the illness and disorder that glycation is responsible for.

The following studies are available on the National Library of Medicine's *PubMed.gov*, out of 11,750 studies at last check.

This study done on glycative effects and Alzheimer's disease was completed in 2005. Glycation of cholesterol into amyloid plaque was researched in this study. It showed that the plaque was responsible for Alzheimer's disease.

Where were the warnings then? It's now 12 years later and millions of people have died from Alzheimer's disease. The question I ask is why? Why weren't we notified of this revelation 14 years ago? It's been in the archives of PubMed since then. Why the delay? How much more must die before this news of the glycative effects of glucose, is publicized so that the FDA and the USDA have to recognize its dangers?

This report from Sep 20, 2005, explains how the plaques from glycation contribute to Alzheimer's disease;

- *5-aminoimidazole-4-carboxamide-1-beta-4-ribofuranoside (AICAR) attenuates the expression of LPS- and Aβ peptide-induced inflammatory mediators in astroglia. J Biol Chem. 1985 Sep 5;260(19):10629-36.*

Alzheimer's disease (AD) pathology shows characteristic 'plaques' rich in amyloid beta (Aβ) peptide deposits. Inflammatory process-related proteins such as pro-inflammatory cytokines have been detected in AD brain suggesting that an inflammatory immune reaction also plays a role in the pathogenesis of AD.
Alzheimer's disease (AD) is a neurological disorder and the brain pathology is characterized by the presence of senile plaques rich in insoluble aggregates of beta-amyloid (1–40) and (1–42) peptides, degradation products of the larger amyloid precursor protein. All major pro-inflammatory cytokines with the exception of IFN-γ (TNF-α, IL-1, and IL-6) have been detected in AD brain suggesting that an inflammatory immune reaction also plays a role in the pathogenesis of AD. The deposited Aβ peptides have also been implicated in oxidative stress-induced responses, via NADPH oxidase activation and superoxide anion generation.

This has been known for more than 11 years, yet nobody knows about it except for a few researchers. Fewer are trying to disseminate this info.

This study done on the effects of glucose on glycation was done in September 1985. Have you seen or heard of any part of this report prior to today? I haven't. I had to search for it. The question I have is why wasn't the public notified of this revelation? Were the research results suppressed so as to hide the truth from the public? I have to wonder.

Glycation of amino groups in protein. Studies on the specificity of modification of RNase by glucose.
Watkins NG, Thorpe SR, Baynes JW.

Ribonuclease A has been used as a model protein for studying
the specificity of glycation of amino groups in protein under physiological
conditions (phosphate buffer, pH 7.4, 37 degrees C). Incubation
of RNase with glucose led to an enhanced rate of inactivation of the enzyme
relative to the rate of modification of lysine residues, suggesting a
preferential modification of active site lysine residues…Both the equilibrium
Schiff base concentration and the rate of the Amadori rearrangement at each
site were found to be important in determining
the specificity of glycation of RNase.

This means that around 1985, they were learning about the effects of glycation, yet an industry that depends on this action to feed their customer base in the pharmaceutical industry, was doing what it could to keep these reports from becoming public information.

About this same time, according to Wikipedia;

IN 1985, MONSANTO ACQUIRED G. D. SEARLE & COMPANY, A LIFE SCIENCES COMPANY FOCUSING ON PHARMACEUTICALS, AGRICULTURE AND ANIMAL HEALTH. IN 1993, ITS SEARLE DIVISION FILED A PATENT APPLICATION FOR CELEBREX, WHICH IN 1998 BECAME THE FIRST SELECTIVE COX-2 INHIBITOR TO BE APPROVED BY THE U.S. FOOD AND DRUG ADMINISTRATION (FDA). CELEBREX BECAME A BLOCK BUSTER DRUG AND WAS OFTEN MENTIONED AS A KEY REASON FOR PFIZER'S ACQUISITION OF MONSANTO'S PHARMACEUTICAL BUSINESS IN 2002.

Was it coincidence? I have to wonder. Since then Monsanto has made moves to control all of the grain industry in America, by contracting farmers to grow no other seed than their own GMO seed. This allows the farmers who do this to spray massive amounts of herbicide on those crops. The herbicide they spray is Monsanto's Roundup, a glyphosate herbicide that works by inhibiting the actions of enzymes. Enzymes are important proteins and peptides in the body as they're cell signaling proteins that instruct cells how to operate. This is important because it's that instruction that the cells need to **not become glycation.**

Otherwise, without that enzyme, you create glycation and inflammation. Inflammation is the foundation of all modern diseases. This is why grains are slowly killing those who eat them, cutting their lives short, to the tune of 2,684 deaths every day can be attributed to these killing field grains. These signaling cells are cells like hormones and polypeptides that affect your body's functions. If these aren't working because of an enzyme inhibitor floating around in your blood, it's going to lead to glycation and disease. This is the scary part of this story if you eat bread or anything flour is used in, you're eating this herbicide along with your bread. If you use canola oil or eat corn chips when you go out for Mexican food, you're putting this glyphosate herbicide in your body. It's used on **ALL** corn products, **ALL** soy products. Monsanto removed GMO wheat seeds from the market due to restrictions on GMO foods in the European market.

This study was completed in September 1985, about the same time Monsanto acquired G.D. Searle Pharmaceuticals. 8 years later they filed for a patent for Celebrex their arthritis painkiller drug. Celebrex is a Cox 2 NSAID with the following side effects and concerns, according to Searle, and I'm listing all of them. (16 pages worth); If you take this drug, read this disclaimer well.

CONTRAINDICATIONS

NSAIDS MAY BE USED WITH CAUTION BY PEOPLE WITH THE FOLLOWING CONDITIONS:

IRRITABLE BOWEL SYNDROME

- *PERSONS WHO ARE OVER AGE 50, AND WHO HAVE A FAMILY HISTORY OF GI (GASTROINTESTINAL) PROBLEMS*
- *PERSONS WHO HAVE HAD PAST GI PROBLEMS FROM NSAID USE*

NSAIDS SHOULD USUALLY BE AVOIDED BY PEOPLE WITH THE FOLLOWING CONDITIONS:

- *PEPTIC ULCER OR STOMACH BLEEDING*
- *UNCONTROLLED HYPERTENSION*
- *KIDNEY DISEASE*
- *PEOPLE THAT SUFFER FROM INFLAMMATORY BOWEL DISEASE (CROHN'S DISEASE OR ULCERATIVE COLITIS)[6]*
- *PAST TRANSIENT ISCHEMIC ATTACK(EXCLUDING IBUPROFEN)*
- *PAST STROKE(EXCLUDING IBUPROFEN)*
- *PAST MYOCARDIAL INFARCTION(EXCLUDING IBUPROFEN)[6]*
- *CORONARY ARTERY DISEASE(EXCLUDING IBUPROFEN)[6]*
- *UNDERGOING CORONARY ARTERY BYPASS SURGERY[6]*
- *TAKING IBUPROFEN FOR HEART*
- *CONGESTIVE HEART FAILURE(EXCLUDING LOW-DOSE IBUPROFEN)*

- *IN THE THIRD TRIMESTER OF PREGNANCY*
- *PERSONS WHO HAVE UNDERGONE GASTRIC BYPASS SURGERY*
- *PERSONS WHO HAVE A HISTORY OF ALLERGIC OR ALLERGIC-TYPE NSAID HYPERSENSITIVITY REACTIONS, E.G. ASPIRIN-INDUCED ASTHMA*

ADVERSE EFFECTS

THE WIDESPREAD USE OF NSAIDS HAS MEANT THAT THE ADVERSE EFFECTS OF THESE DRUGS HAVE BECOME INCREASINGLY COMMON. USE OF NSAIDS INCREASES RISK OF HAVING A RANGE OF GASTROINTESTINAL(GI) PROBLEMS. WHEN NSAIDS ARE USED FOR PAIN MANAGEMENT AFTER SURGERY THEY CAUSE INCREASED RISK OF KIDNEY PROBLEMS. AN ESTIMATED 10–20% OF NSAID PATIENTS EXPERIENCE DYSPEPSIA. IN THE 1990S HIGH DOSES OF PRESCRIPTION NSAIDS WERE ASSOCIATED WITH SERIOUS UPPER GASTROINTESTINAL ADVERSE EVENTS, INCLUDING BLEEDING. OVER THE PAST DECADE, DEATHS ASSOCIATED WITH GASTRIC BLEEDING HAVE DECLINED.

NSAIDS, LIKE ALL DRUGS, MAY INTERACT WITH OTHER MEDICATIONS. FOR EXAMPLE, CONCURRENT USE OF NSAIDS AND QUINOLONES MAY INCREASE THE RISK OF QUINOLONES' ADVERSE CENTRAL NERVOUS SYSTEM EFFECTS, INCLUDING SEIZURE.

THERE IS ARGUMENT OVER THE BENEFITS AND RISKS OF NSAIDS FOR TREATING CHRONIC MUSCULOSKELETAL PAIN. EACH DRUG HAS A BENEFIT-RISK PROFILE AND BALANCING THE RISK OF NO TREATMENT WITH THE COMPETING POTENTIAL RISKS OF VARIOUS THERAPIES IS THE CLINICIAN'S RESPONSIBILITY.

COMBINATIONAL RISK

IF A COX-2 INHIBITOR IS TAKEN, A TRADITIONAL NSAID (PRESCRIPTION OR OVER-THE-COUNTER) SHOULD NOT BE TAKEN AT THE SAME TIME. IN ADDITION, PEOPLE ON DAILY ASPIRIN THERAPY (E.G., FOR REDUCING CARDIOVASCULAR RISK) MUST BE CAREFUL IF THEY ALSO USE OTHER NSAIDS, AS THESE MAY INHIBIT THE CARDIOPROTECTIVE EFFECTS OF ASPIRIN.

ROFECOXIB (VIOXX) WAS SHOWN TO PRODUCE SIGNIFICANTLY FEWER GASTROINTESTINAL ADVERSE DRUG REACTIONS (ADRS) COMPARED WITH NAPROXEN. THIS STUDY, THE VIGOR TRIAL, RAISED THE ISSUE OF THE CARDIOVASCULAR SAFETY OF THE COXIBS. A STATISTICALLY SIGNIFICANT INCREASE IN THE INCIDENCE OF MYOCARDIAL INFARCTIONS WAS OBSERVED IN PATIENTS ON ROFECOXIB. FURTHER DATA, FROM THE APPROVE TRIAL, SHOWED A STATISTICALLY SIGNIFICANT RELATIVE RISK OF CARDIOVASCULAR EVENTS OF 1.97 VERSUS PLACEBO WHICH CAUSED A WORLDWIDE WITHDRAWAL OF ROFECOXIB IN OCTOBER 2004.

USE OF METHOTREXATE TOGETHER WITH NSAIDS IN RHEUMATOID ARTHRITIS IS SAFE IF ADEQUATE MONITORING IS DONE.

CARDIOVASCULAR

NSAIDS ASIDE FROM ASPIRIN, BOTH NEWER SELECTIVE COX-2 INHIBITORS AND TRADITIONAL ANTI-INFLAMMATORIES, INCREASE THE RISK OF MYOCARDIAL INFARCTION AND STROKE. THEY ARE NOT RECOMMENDED IN THOSE WHO HAVE HAD A PREVIOUS HEART ATTACK AS THEY INCREASE THE RISK OF DEATH AND/OR RECURRENT MI. EVIDENCE INDICATES THAT NAPROXEN MAY BE THE LEAST HARMFUL OUT OF THESE.

NSAIDS ASIDE FROM (LOW-DOSE) ASPIRIN ARE ASSOCIATED WITH A DOUBLED RISK OF HEART FAILURE IN PEOPLE WITHOUT A HISTORY OF CARDIAC DISEASE. IN PEOPLE WITH SUCH A HISTORY, USE OF NSAIDS (ASIDE FROM LOW-DOSE ASPIRIN) WAS ASSOCIATED WITH A MORE THAN 10-FOLD INCREASE IN HEART FAILURE. IF THIS LINK IS PROVEN CAUSAL, RESEARCHERS ESTIMATE THAT NSAIDS WOULD BE RESPONSIBLE FOR UP TO 20 PERCENT OF HOSPITAL ADMISSIONS FOR CONGESTIVE HEART FAILURE. IN PEOPLE WITH HEART FAILURE, NSAIDS INCREASE MORTALITY RISK (HAZARD RATIO) BY APPROXIMATELY 1.2–1.3 FOR NAPROXEN AND IBUPROFEN, 1.7 FOR ROFECOXIB AND CELECOXIB, AND 2.1 FOR DICLOFENAC.

ON 9 JULY 2015, THE FDA TOUGHENED WARNINGS OF INCREASED HEART ATTACK AND STROKE RISK ASSOCIATED WITH NONSTEROIDAL ANTI-INFLAMMATORY DRUGS (NSAID). ASPIRIN IS AN NSAID BUT IS NOT AFFECTED BY THE NEW WARNINGS.

POSSIBLE ERECTILE DYSFUNCTION RISK

A 2005 FINNISH STUDY LINKED LONG TERM (OVER 3 MONTHS) USE OF NSAIDS WITH AN INCREASED RISK OF ERECTILE DYSFUNCTION. THIS STUDY WAS CORRELATIONAL ONLY AND DEPENDED SOLELY ON SELF-REPORTS (QUESTIONNAIRES).

A 2011 PUBLICATION IN THE JOURNAL OF UROLOGY RECEIVED WIDESPREAD PUBLICITY. ACCORDING TO THIS STUDY, MEN WHO USED NSAIDS REGULARLY WERE AT SIGNIFICANTLY INCREASED RISK OF ERECTILE DYSFUNCTION. A LINK BETWEEN NSAID USE AND ERECTILE DYSFUNCTION STILL EXISTED AFTER CONTROLLING FOR SEVERAL CONDITIONS. HOWEVER, THE STUDY WAS OBSERVATIONAL AND NOT CONTROLLED, WITH LOW ORIGINAL PARTICIPATION RATE, POTENTIAL PARTICIPATION BIAS, AND OTHER UNCONTROLLED FACTORS. THE AUTHORS WARNED AGAINST DRAWING ANY CONCLUSION REGARDING CAUSE.

GASTROINTESTINAL

THE MAIN ADVERSE DRUG REACTIONS (ADRS) ASSOCIATED WITH NSAID USE RELATE TO DIRECT AND INDIRECT IRRITATION OF THE GASTROINTESTINAL (GI) TRACT. NSAIDS CAUSE A DUAL ASSAULT ON THE GI TRACT: THE ACIDIC MOLECULES DIRECTLY IRRITATE THE GASTRIC MUCOSA, AND INHIBITION OF COX-1 AND COX-2 REDUCES THE LEVELS OF PROTECTIVE PROSTAGLANDINS. INHIBITION OF PROSTAGLANDIN SYNTHESIS IN THE GI TRACT CAUSES INCREASED GASTRIC ACID SECRETION, DIMINISHED BICARBONATE SECRETION, DIMINISHED MUCUS SECRETION AND DIMINISHED TROPHIC [EFFECTS ON EPITHELIAL MUCOSA. COMMON GASTROINTESTINAL ADRS INCLUDE

- NAUSEA/VOMITING
- DYSPEPSIA
- GASTRIC ULCERATION/BLEEDING
- DIARRHEA

CLINICAL NSAID ULCERS ARE RELATED TO THE SYSTEMIC EFFECTS OF NSAID ADMINISTRATION. SUCH DAMAGE OCCURS IRRESPECTIVE OF THE ROUTE OF ADMINISTRATION OF THE NSAID (E.G., ORAL, RECTAL, OR PARENTERAL) AND CAN OCCUR EVEN IN PATIENTS WITH ACHLORHYDRIA.

ULCERATION RISK INCREASES WITH THERAPY DURATION, AND WITH HIGHER DOSES. TO MINIMISE GI ADRS, IT IS PRUDENT TO USE THE LOWEST EFFECTIVE DOSE FOR THE SHORTEST PERIOD OF TIME—A PRACTICE THAT STUDIES SHOW IS OFTEN NOT FOLLOWED. RECENT STUDIES SHOW THAT OVER 50% OF PATIENTS WHO TAKE NSAIDS HAVE SUSTAINED SOME MUCOSAL DAMAGE TO THEIR SMALL INTESTINE.

THERE ARE ALSO SOME DIFFERENCES IN THE PROPENSITY OF INDIVIDUAL AGENTS TO CAUSE GASTROINTESTINAL ADRS. INDOMETHACIN, KETOPROFEN, AND PIROXICAM APPEAR TO HAVE THE HIGHEST PREVALENCE OF GASTRIC ADRS, WHILE IBUPROFEN (LOWER DOSES) AND DICLOFENAC, APPEAR TO HAVE LOWER RATES.

CERTAIN NSAIDS, SUCH AS ASPIRIN, HAVE BEEN MARKETED IN ENTERIC-COATED FORMULATIONS THAT MANUFACTURERS CLAIM REDUCE THE INCIDENCE OF GASTROINTESTINAL ADRS. SIMILARLY, SOME BELIEVE THAT RECTAL FORMULATIONS MAY REDUCE GASTROINTESTINAL ADRS. HOWEVER, CONSISTENT WITH THE SYSTEMIC MECHANISM OF SUCH ADRS, AND IN CLINICAL PRACTICE, THESE FORMULATIONS HAVE NOT DEMONSTRATED A REDUCED RISK OF GI ULCERATION.

COMMONLY, GASTRIC (BUT NOT NECESSARILY INTESTINAL) ADVERSE EFFECTS CAN BE REDUCED THROUGH SUPPRESSING ACID PRODUCTION, BY CONCOMITANT USE OF A PROTON PUMP INHIBITOR, E.G., OMEPRAZOLE, ESOMEPRAZOLE; OR THE PROSTAGLANDIN ANALOGUE MISOPROSTOL. MISOPROSTOL IS ITSELF ASSOCIATED WITH A HIGH INCIDENCE OF GASTROINTESTINAL ADRS (DIARRHEA). WHILE THESE TECHNIQUES MAY BE EFFECTIVE, THEY ARE EXPENSIVE FOR MAINTENANCE THERAPY.

INFLAMMATORY BOWEL DISEASE

NSAIDS SHOULD BE USED WITH CAUTION IN INDIVIDUALS WITH INFLAMMATORY BOWEL DISEASE (E.G., CROHN'S DISEASE OR ULCERATIVE COLITIS) DUE TO THEIR TENDENCY TO CAUSE GASTRIC BLEEDING AND FORM ULCERATION IN THE GASTRIC LINING. PAIN RELIEVERS SUCH AS PARACETAMOL (ALSO KNOWN AS ACETAMINOPHEN) OR DRUGS CONTAINING CODEINE (WHICH

SLOWS DOWN BOWEL ACTIVITY) ARE SAFER MEDICATIONS FOR PAIN RELIEF IN IBD.

RENAL

NSAIDS ARE ALSO ASSOCIATED WITH A FAIRLY HIGH INCIDENCE OF RENAL ADVERSE DRUG REACTIONS (ADRS). THE MECHANISM OF THESE RENAL ADRS IS DUE TO CHANGES IN RENAL HAEMODYNAMICS (KIDNEY BLOOD FLOW), ORDINARILY MEDIATED BY PROSTAGLANDINS, WHICH ARE AFFECTED BY NSAIDS. PROSTAGLANDINS NORMALLY CAUSE VASODILATION OF THE AFFERENT ARTERIOLES OF THE GLOMERULI. THIS HELPS MAINTAIN NORMAL GLOMERULAR PERFUSION AND GLOMERULAR FILTRATION RATE (GFR), AN INDICATOR OF RENAL FUNCTION. THIS IS PARTICULARLY IMPORTANT IN RENAL FAILURE WHERE THE KIDNEY IS TRYING TO MAINTAIN RENAL PERFUSION PRESSURE BY ELEVATED ANGIOTENSIN II LEVELS. AT THESE ELEVATED LEVELS, ANGIOTENSIN II ALSO CONSTRICTS THE AFFERENT ARTERIOLE INTO THE GLOMERULUS IN ADDITION TO THE EFFERENT ARTERIOLE IT NORMALLY CONSTRICTS. PROSTAGLANDINS SERVE TO DILATE THE AFFERENT ARTERIOLE; BY BLOCKING THIS PROSTAGLANDIN-MEDIATED EFFECT, PARTICULARLY IN RENAL FAILURE, NSAIDS CAUSE UNOPPOSED CONSTRICTION OF THE AFFERENT ARTERIOLE AND DECREASED RPF (RENAL PERFUSION PRESSURE).

COMMON ADRS ASSOCIATED WITH ALTERED RENAL FUNCTION INCLUDE:

- *SALT (SODIUM) AND FLUID RETENTION*
- *HYPERTENSION(HIGH BLOOD PRESSURE)*

THESE AGENTS MAY ALSO CAUSE RENAL IMPAIRMENT, ESPECIALLY IN COMBINATION WITH OTHER NEPHROTOXIC AGENTS. RENAL FAILURE IS ESPECIALLY A RISK IF THE PATIENT IS ALSO CONCOMITANTLY TAKING AN ACE INHIBITOR (WHICH REMOVES ANGIOTENSIN II'S VASOCONSTRICTION OF THE EFFERENT ARTERIOLE) AND A DIURETIC (WHICH DROPS PLASMA VOLUME, AND THEREBY RPF)—THE SO-CALLED "TRIPLE WHAMMY" EFFECT.

IN RARER INSTANCES NSAIDS MAY ALSO CAUSE MORE SEVERE RENAL CONDITIONS:

- *INTERSTITIAL NEPHRITIS*

- *NEPHROTIC SYNDROME*
- *ACUTE RENAL FAILURE*
- *ACUTE TUBULAR NECROSIS*
- *RENAL PAPILLARY NECROSIS*

NSAIDS IN COMBINATION WITH EXCESSIVE USE OF PHENACETINAND/OR PARACETAMOL (ACETAMINOPHEN) MAY LEAD TO ANALGESIC NEPHROPATHY.

PHOTOSENSITIVITY

PHOTOSENSITIVITY IS A COMMONLY OVERLOOKED ADVERSE EFFECT OF MANY OF THE NSAIDS. THE 2-ARYLPROPIONIC ACIDS ARE THE MOST LIKELY TO PRODUCE PHOTOSENSITIVITY REACTIONS, BUT OTHER NSAIDS HAVE ALSO BEEN IMPLICATED INCLUDING PIROXICAM, DICLOFENAC, AND BENZYDAMINE.

BENOXAPROFEN, SINCE WITHDRAWN DUE TO ITS HEPATOTOXICITY, WAS THE MOST PHOTOACTIVE NSAID OBSERVED. THE MECHANISM OF PHOTOSENSITIVITY, RESPONSIBLE FOR THE HIGH PHOTOACTIVITY OF THE 2-ARYLPROPIONIC ACIDS, IS THE READY DECARBOXYLATION OF THE CARBOXYLIC ACID MOIETY. THE SPECIFIC ABSORBANCE CHARACTERISTICS OF THE DIFFERENT CHROMOPHORIC 2-ARYL SUBSTITUENTS, AFFECTS THE DECARBOXYLATION MECHANISM. WHILE IBUPROFEN HAS WEAK ABSORPTION, IT HAS BEEN REPORTED AS A WEAK PHOTOSENSITISING AGENT.

DURING PREGNANCY

NSAIDS ARE NOT RECOMMENDED DURING PREGNANCY, PARTICULARLY DURING THE THIRD TRIMESTER. WHILE NSAIDS AS A CLASS IS NOT DIRECT TERATOGENS, THEY MAY CAUSE PREMATURE CLOSURE OF THE FETAL DUCTUS ARTERIOSUS AND RENAL ADRS IN THE FETUS. ADDITIONALLY, THEY ARE LINKED WITH PREMATURE BIRTH AND MISCARRIAGE. ASPIRIN, HOWEVER, IS USED TOGETHER WITH HEPARIN IN PREGNANT WOMEN WITH ANTIPHOSPHOLIPID ANTIBODIES. ADDITIONALLY, INDOMETHACIN IS USED IN PREGNANCY TO TREAT POLYHYDRAMNIOS BY REDUCING FETAL URINE PRODUCTION VIA INHIBITING FETAL RENAL BLOOD FLOW.

IN CONTRAST, PARACETAMOL (ACETAMINOPHEN) IS REGARDED AS BEING SAFE AND WELL-TOLERATED DURING PREGNANCY, BUT LEFFERS ET AL. RELEASED A STUDY IN 2010 INDICATING THAT THERE MAY BE ASSOCIATED MALE INFERTILITY IN THE UNBORN. DOSES SHOULD BE TAKEN AS PRESCRIBED, DUE TO RISK OF HEPATOTOXICITY WITH OVERDOSES. IN FRANCE, THE COUNTRY'S HEALTH AGENCY CONTRAINDICATES THE USE OF NSAIDS, INCLUDING ASPIRIN, AFTER THE SIXTH MONTH OF PREGNANCY.

ALLERGY/ALLERGY-LIKE HYPERSENSITIVITY REACTIONS

A VARIETY OF ALLERGIC OR ALLERGIC-LIKE NSAID HYPERSENSITIVITY REACTIONS FOLLOW THE INGESTION OF NSAIDS. THESE HYPERSENSITIVITY REACTIONS DIFFER FROM THE OTHER ADVERSE REACTIONS LISTED HERE WHICH ARE TOXICITY REACTIONS, I.E. UNWANTED REACTIONS THAT RESULT FROM THE PHARMACOLOGICAL ACTION OF A DRUG, ARE DOSE-RELATED, AND CAN OCCUR IN ANY TREATED INDIVIDUAL; HYPERSENSITIVITY REACTIONS ARE IDIOSYNCRATIC REACTIONS TO A DRUG.[51] SOME NSAID HYPERSENSITIVITY REACTIONS ARE TRULY ALLERGIC IN ORIGIN: *1)* REPETITIVE IGE-MEDIATED URTICARIAL SKIN ERUPTIONS, ANGIOEDEMA, AND ANAPHYLAXIS FOLLOWING IMMEDIATELY TO HOURS AFTER INGESTING ONE STRUCTURAL TYPE OF NSAID BUT NOT AFTER INGESTING STRUCTURALLY UNRELATED NSAIDS; AND *2)*COMPARATIVELY MILD TO MODERATELY SEVERE T CELL-MEDIATED DELAYED ONSET (USUALLY MORE THAN 24 HOUR), SKIN REACTIONS SUCH AS MACULOPAPULAR RASH, FIXED DRUG ERUPTIONS, PHOTOSENSITIVITY REACTIONS, DELAYED URTICARIA, AND CONTACT DERMATITIS; OR *3)* FAR MORE SEVERE AND POTENTIALLY LIFE-THREATENING T-CELL MEDIATED DELAYED SYSTEMIC REACTIONS SUCH AS THE DRESS SYNDROME, ACUTE GENERALIZED EXANTHEMATOUS PUSTULOSIS, THE STEVENS–JOHNSON SYNDROME, AND TOXIC EPIDERMAL NECROLYSIS. OTHER NSAID HYPERSENSITIVITY REACTIONS ARE ALLERGY-LIKE SYMPTOMS BUT DO NOT INVOLVE TRUE ALLERGIC MECHANISMS; RATHER, THEY APPEAR DUE TO THE ABILITY OF NSAIDS TO ALTER THE METABOLISM OF ARACHIDONIC ACID IN FAVOR OF FORMING METABOLITES THAT PROMOTE ALLERGIC SYMPTOMS. AFFLICTED INDIVIDUALS MAY BE ABNORMALLY SENSITIVE TO THESE PROVOCATIVE METABOLITES AND/OR OVERPRODUCE THEM AND TYPICALLY ARE SUSCEPTIBLE TO A WIDE RANGE OF

STRUCTURALLY DISSIMILAR NSAIDS, PARTICULARLY THOSE THAT INHIBIT COX1. SYMPTOMS, WHICH DEVELOP IMMEDIATELY TO HOURS AFTER INGESTING ANY OF VARIOUS NSAIDS THAT INHIBIT COX-1, ARE: **1)**EXACERBATIONS OF ASTHMATIC AND RHINITIS (SEE ASPIRIN-INDUCED ASTHMA) SYMPTOMS IN INDIVIDUALS WITH A HISTORY OF ASTHMA OR RHINITIS AND **2)** EXACERBATION OR FIRST-TIME DEVELOPMENT OF WHEALS AND/OR ANGIOEDEMA IN INDIVIDUALS WITH OR WITHOUT A HISTORY OF CHRONIC URTICARIAL LESIONS OR ANGIOEDEMA.

CONTRAINDICATIONS

NSAIDS MAY BE USED WITH CAUTION BY PEOPLE WITH THE FOLLOWING CONDITIONS

- IRRITABLE BOWEL SYNDROME
- PERSONS WHO ARE OVER AGE 50, AND WHO HAVE A FAMILY HISTORY OF GI (GASTROINTESTINAL) PROBLEMS
- PERSONS WHO HAVE HAD PAST GI PROBLEMS FROM NSAID USE

NSAIDS SHOULD USUALLY BE AVOIDED BY PEOPLE WITH THE FOLLOWING CONDITIONS

- PEPTIC ULCER OR STOMACH BLEEDING
- UNCONTROLLED HYPERTENSION
- KIDNEY DISEASE
- PEOPLE THAT SUFFER FROM INFLAMMATORY BOWEL DISEASE (CROHN'S DISEASE OR ULCERATIVE COLITIS)
- PAST TRANSIENT ISCHEMIC ATTACK (EXCLUDING IBUPROFEN)
- PAST STROKE (EXCLUDING IBUPROFEN)
- PAST MYOCARDIAL INFARCTION (EXCLUDING IBUPROFEN)
- CORONARY ARTERY DISEASE(EXCLUDING IBUPROFEN)]
- UNDERGOING CORONARY ARTERY BYPASS SURGERY
- TAKING IBUPROFEN FOR HEART
- CONGESTIVE HEART FAILURE(EXCLUDING LOW-DOSE IBUPROFEN)
- IN THE THIRD TRIMESTER OF PREGNANCY
- PERSONS WHO HAVE UNDERGONE GASTRIC BYPASS SURGERY

- *PERSONS WHO HAVE A HISTORY OF ALLERGIC OR ALLERGIC-TYPE NSAID HYPERSENSITIVITY REACTIONS, E.G. ASPIRIN-INDUCED ASTHMA*

ADVERSE EFFECTS

THE WIDESPREAD USE OF NSAIDS HAS MEANT THAT THE ADVERSE EFFECTS OF THESE DRUGS HAVE BECOME INCREASINGLY COMMON. USE OF NSAIDS INCREASES RISK OF HAVING A RANGE OF GASTROINTESTINAL(GI) PROBLEMS. WHEN NSAIDS ARE USED FOR PAIN MANAGEMENT AFTER SURGERY THEY CAUSE INCREASED RISK OF KIDNEY PROBLEMS.

AN ESTIMATED 10–20% OF NSAID PATIENTS EXPERIENCE DYSPEPSIA. IN THE 1990S HIGH DOSES OF PRESCRIPTION NSAIDS WERE ASSOCIATED WITH SERIOUS UPPER GASTROINTESTINAL ADVERSE EVENTS, INCLUDING BLEEDING. OVER THE PAST DECADE, DEATHS ASSOCIATED WITH GASTRIC BLEEDING HAVE DECLINED.

NSAIDS, LIKE ALL DRUGS, MAY INTERACT WITH OTHER MEDICATIONS. FOR EXAMPLE, CONCURRENT USE OF NSAIDS AND QUINOLONES MAY INCREASE THE RISK OF QUINOLONES' ADVERSE CENTRAL NERVOUS SYSTEM EFFECTS, INCLUDING SEIZURE.

THERE IS ARGUMENT OVER THE BENEFITS AND RISKS OF NSAIDS FOR TREATING CHRONIC MUSCULOSKELETAL PAIN. EACH DRUG HAS A BENEFIT-RISK PROFILE AND BALANCING THE RISK OF NO TREATMENT WITH THE COMPETING POTENTIAL RISKS OF VARIOUS THERAPIES IS THE CLINICIAN'S RESPONSIBILITY.

COMBINATIONAL RISK

IF A COX-2 INHIBITOR IS TAKEN, A TRADITIONAL NSAID (PRESCRIPTION OR OVER-THE-COUNTER) SHOULD NOT BE TAKEN AT THE SAME TIME. IN ADDITION, PEOPLE ON DAILY ASPIRIN THERAPY (E.G., FOR REDUCING CARDIOVASCULAR RISK) MUST BE CAREFUL IF THEY ALSO USE OTHER NSAIDS, AS THESE MAY INHIBIT THE CARDIOPROTECTIVE EFFECTS OF ASPIRIN.

ROFECOXIB (VIOXX) WAS SHOWN TO PRODUCE SIGNIFICANTLY FEWER GASTROINTESTINAL ADVERSE DRUG REACTIONS (ADRS) COMPARED WITH NAPROXEN. THIS STUDY, THE VIGOR TRIAL, RAISED THE ISSUE OF THE CARDIOVASCULAR SAFETY OF THE COXIBS. A STATISTICALLY SIGNIFICANT INCREASE IN THE

INCIDENCE OF MYOCARDIAL INFARCTIONS WAS OBSERVED IN PATIENTS ON ROFECOXIB. FURTHER DATA, FROM THE APPROVE TRIAL, SHOWED A STATISTICALLY SIGNIFICANT RELATIVE RISK OF CARDIOVASCULAR EVENTS OF 1.97 VERSUS PLACEBO WHICH CAUSED A WORLDWIDE WITHDRAWAL OF ROFECOXIB IN OCTOBER 2004.

USE OF METHOTREXATE TOGETHER WITH NSAIDS IN RHEUMATOID ARTHRITIS IS SAFE IF ADEQUATE MONITORING IS DONE.

CARDIOVASCULAR

NSAIDS ASIDE FROM ASPIRIN, BOTH NEWER SELECTIVE COX-2 INHIBITORS AND TRADITIONAL ANTI-INFLAMMATORIES, INCREASE THE RISK OF MYOCARDIAL INFARCTION AND STROKE. THEY ARE NOT RECOMMENDED IN THOSE WHO HAVE HAD A PREVIOUS HEART ATTACK AS THEY INCREASE THE RISK OF DEATH AND/OR RECURRENT MI. EVIDENCE INDICATES THAT NAPROXEN MAY BE THE LEAST HARMFUL OUT OF THESE.

NSAIDS ASIDE FROM (LOW-DOSE) ASPIRIN ARE ASSOCIATED WITH A DOUBLED RISK OF HEART FAILURE IN PEOPLE WITHOUT A HISTORY OF CARDIAC DISEASE. IN PEOPLE WITH SUCH A HISTORY, USE OF NSAIDS (ASIDE FROM LOW-DOSE ASPIRIN) WAS ASSOCIATED WITH A MORE THAN 10-FOLD INCREASE IN HEART FAILURE. IF THIS LINK IS PROVEN CAUSAL, RESEARCHERS ESTIMATE THAT NSAIDS WOULD BE RESPONSIBLE FOR UP TO 20 PERCENT OF HOSPITAL ADMISSIONS FOR CONGESTIVE HEART FAILURE. IN PEOPLE WITH HEART FAILURE, NSAIDS INCREASE MORTALITY RISK (HAZARD RATIO) BY APPROXIMATELY 1.2–1.3 FOR NAPROXEN AND IBUPROFEN, 1.7 FOR ROFECOXIB AND CELECOXIB, AND 2.1 FOR DICLOFENAC.

ON 9 JULY 2015, THE FDA TOUGHENED WARNINGS OF INCREASED HEART ATTACK AND STROKE RISK ASSOCIATED WITH NONSTEROIDAL ANTI-INFLAMMATORY DRUGS (NSAID). ASPIRIN IS AN NSAID BUT IS NOT AFFECTED BY THE NEW WARNINGS.

POSSIBLE ERECTILE DYSFUNCTION RISK

A 2005 FINNISH STUDY LINKED LONG TERM (OVER 3 MONTHS) USE OF NSAIDS WITH AN INCREASED RISK OF ERECTILE DYSFUNCTION. THIS STUDY WAS CORRELATIONAL ONLY AND DEPENDED SOLELY ON SELF-REPORTS (QUESTIONNAIRES).

A 2011 PUBLICATION IN THE JOURNAL OF UROLOGY RECEIVED WIDESPREAD PUBLICITY. ACCORDING TO THIS STUDY, MEN WHO USED NSAIDS REGULARLY WERE AT SIGNIFICANTLY INCREASED RISK OF ERECTILE DYSFUNCTION. A LINK BETWEEN NSAID USE AND ERECTILE DYSFUNCTION STILL EXISTED AFTER CONTROLLING FOR SEVERAL CONDITIONS. HOWEVER, THE STUDY WAS OBSERVATIONAL AND NOT CONTROLLED, WITH LOW ORIGINAL PARTICIPATION RATE, POTENTIAL PARTICIPATION BIAS, AND OTHER UNCONTROLLED FACTORS. THE AUTHORS WARNED AGAINST DRAWING ANY CONCLUSION REGARDING CAUSE.

GASTROINTESTINAL

THE MAIN ADVERSE DRUG REACTIONS (ADRS) ASSOCIATED WITH NSAID USE RELATE TO DIRECT AND INDIRECT IRRITATION OF THE GASTROINTESTINAL (GI) TRACT. NSAIDS CAUSE A DUAL ASSAULT ON THE GI TRACT: THE ACIDIC MOLECULES DIRECTLY IRRITATE THE GASTRIC MUCOSA, AND INHIBITION OF COX-1 AND COX-2 REDUCES THE LEVELS OF PROTECTIVE PROSTAGLANDINS. INHIBITION OF PROSTAGLANDIN SYNTHESIS IN THE GI TRACT CAUSES INCREASED GASTRIC ACID SECRETION, DIMINISHED BICARBONATE SECRETION, DIMINISHED MUCUS SECRETION AND DIMINISHED TROPHIC EFFECTS ON EPITHELIAL MUCOSA.

COMMON GASTROINTESTINAL ADRS INCLUDE:

- *NAUSEA/VOMITING*
- *DYSPEPSIA*
- *GASTRIC ULCERATION/BLEEDING*
- *DIARRHEA*

CLINICAL NSAID ULCERS ARE RELATED TO THE SYSTEMIC EFFECTS OF NSAID ADMINISTRATION. SUCH DAMAGE OCCURS IRRESPECTIVE OF THE ROUTE OF ADMINISTRATION OF THE NSAID (E.G., ORAL, RECTAL, OR PARENTERAL) AND CAN OCCUR EVEN IN PATIENTS WITH ACHLORHYDRIA."

ULCERATION RISK INCREASES WITH THERAPY DURATION, AND WITH HIGHER DOSES. TO MINIMISE GI ADRS, IT IS PRUDENT TO USE THE LOWEST EFFECTIVE DOSE FOR THE SHORTEST PERIOD OF TIME—A PRACTICE THAT STUDIES SHOW IS OFTEN NOT FOLLOWED. RECENT STUDIES SHOW THAT OVER 50% OF PATIENTS WHO TAKE NSAIDS HAVE SUSTAINED SOME MUCOSAL DAMAGE TO THEIR SMALL INTESTINE.

THERE ARE ALSO SOME DIFFERENCES IN THE PROPENSITY OF INDIVIDUAL AGENTS TO CAUSE GASTROINTESTINAL ADRS. INDOMETHACIN, KETOPROFEN, AND PIROXICAM APPEAR TO HAVE THE HIGHEST PREVALENCE OF GASTRIC ADRS, WHILE IBUPROFEN (LOWER DOSES) AND DICLOFENAC, APPEAR TO HAVE LOWER RATES.

CERTAIN NSAIDS, SUCH AS ASPIRIN, HAVE BEEN MARKETED IN ENTERIC-COATED FORMULATIONS THAT MANUFACTURERS CLAIM REDUCE THE INCIDENCE OF GASTROINTESTINAL ADRS. SIMILARLY, SOME BELIEVE THAT RECTAL FORMULATIONS MAY REDUCE GASTROINTESTINAL ADRS. HOWEVER, CONSISTENT WITH THE SYSTEMIC MECHANISM OF SUCH ADRS, AND IN CLINICAL PRACTICE, THESE FORMULATIONS HAVE NOT DEMONSTRATED A REDUCED RISK OF GI ULCERATION.

COMMONLY, GASTRIC (BUT NOT NECESSARILY INTESTINAL) ADVERSE EFFECTS CAN BE REDUCED THROUGH SUPPRESSING ACID PRODUCTION, BY CONCOMITANT USE OF A PROTON PUMP INHIBITOR, E.G., OMEPRAZOLE, ESOMEPRAZOLE; OR THE PROSTAGLANDIN ANALOGUE MISOPROSTOL. MISOPROSTOL IS ITSELF ASSOCIATED WITH A HIGH INCIDENCE OF GASTROINTESTINAL ADRS (DIARRHEA). WHILE THESE TECHNIQUES MAY BE EFFECTIVE, THEY ARE EXPENSIVE FOR MAINTENANCE THERAPY.

INFLAMMATORY BOWEL DISEASE

NSAIDS SHOULD BE USED WITH CAUTION IN INDIVIDUALS WITH INFLAMMATORY BOWEL DISEASE (E.G., **Crohn's disease** OR ULCERATIVE COLITIS) DUE TO THEIR TENDENCY TO CAUSE GASTRIC BLEEDING AND FORM ULCERATION IN THE GASTRIC LINING. PAIN RELIEVERS SUCH AS PARACETAMOL (ALSO KNOWN AS ACETAMINOPHEN) OR DRUGS CONTAINING CODEINE (WHICH SLOWS DOWN BOWEL ACTIVITY) ARE SAFER MEDICATIONS FOR PAIN RELIEF IN IBD.

RENAL

NSAIDS ARE ALSO ASSOCIATED WITH A FAIRLY HIGH INCIDENCE OF RENAL ADVERSE DRUG REACTIONS (ADRS). THE MECHANISM OF THESE RENAL ADRS IS DUE TO CHANGES IN RENAL HAEMODYNAMICS (KIDNEY BLOOD FLOW), ORDINARILY MEDIATED BY PROSTAGLANDINS, WHICH ARE AFFECTED BY NSAIDS. PROSTAGLANDINS NORMALLY CAUSE VASODILATION OF THE AFFERENT ARTERIOLES OF THE GLOMERULI. THIS HELPS

MAINTAIN NORMAL GLOMERULAR PERFUSION AND GLOMERULAR FILTRATION RATE (GFR), AN INDICATOR OF RENAL FUNCTION. THIS IS PARTICULARLY IMPORTANT IN RENAL FAILURE WHERE THE KIDNEY IS TRYING TO MAINTAIN RENAL PERFUSION PRESSURE BY ELEVATED ANGIOTENSIN II LEVELS. AT THESE ELEVATED LEVELS, ANGIOTENSIN II ALSO CONSTRICTS THE AFFERENT ARTERIOLE INTO THE GLOMERULUS IN ADDITION TO THE EFFERENT ARTERIOLE IT NORMALLY CONSTRICTS. PROSTAGLANDINS SERVE TO DILATE THE AFFERENT ARTERIOLE; BY BLOCKING THIS PROSTAGLANDIN-MEDIATED EFFECT, PARTICULARLY IN RENAL FAILURE, NSAIDS CAUSE UNOPPOSED CONSTRICTION OF THE AFFERENT ARTERIOLE AND DECREASED RPF (RENAL PERFUSION PRESSURE). COMMON ADRS ASSOCIATED WITH ALTERED RENAL FUNCTION INCLUDE:

- SALT (SODIUM) AND FLUID RETENTION
- HYPERTENSION(HIGH BLOOD PRESSURE)

THESE AGENTS MAY ALSO CAUSE RENAL IMPAIRMENT, ESPECIALLY IN COMBINATION WITH OTHER NEPHROTOXIC AGENTS. RENAL FAILURE IS ESPECIALLY A RISK IF THE PATIENT IS ALSO CONCOMITANTLY TAKING AN ACE INHIBITOR (WHICH REMOVES ANGIOTENSIN II'S VASOCONSTRICTION OF THE EFFERENT ARTERIOLE) AND A DIURETIC (WHICH DROPS PLASMA VOLUME, AND THEREBY RPF)—THE SO-CALLED "TRIPLE WHAMMY" EFFECT.

IN RARER INSTANCES NSAIDS MAY ALSO CAUSE MORE SEVERE RENAL CONDITIONS:

- INTERSTITIAL NEPHRITIS
- NEPHROTIC SYNDROME
- ACUTE RENAL FAILURE
- ACUTE TUBULAR NECROSIS
- RENAL PAPILLARY NECROSIS

NSAIDS IN COMBINATION WITH EXCESSIVE USE OF PHENACETINAND/OR PARACETAMOL (ACETAMINOPHEN) MAY LEAD TO ANALGESIC NEPHROPATHY.

PHOTOSENSITIVITY

PHOTOSENSITIVITY IS A COMMONLY OVERLOOKED ADVERSE EFFECT OF MANY OF THE NSAIDS. THE 2-ARYLPROPIONIC ACIDS ARE THE MOST LIKELY TO PRODUCE PHOTOSENSITIVITY REACTIONS, BUT OTHER NSAIDS HAVE ALSO BEEN IMPLICATED INCLUDING PIROXICAM, DICLOFENAC, AND BENZYDAMINE.

BENOXAPROFEN, SINCE WITHDRAWN DUE TO ITS HEPATOTOXICITY, WAS THE MOST PHOTOACTIVE NSAID OBSERVED. THE MECHANISM OF PHOTOSENSITIVITY, RESPONSIBLE FOR THE HIGH PHOTOACTIVITY OF THE 2-ARYLPROPIONIC ACIDS, IS THE READY DECARBOXYLATION OF THE CARBOXYLIC ACID MOIETY. THE SPECIFIC ABSORBANCE CHARACTERISTICS OF THE DIFFERENT CHROMOPHORIC 2-ARYL SUBSTITUENTS, AFFECTS THE DECARBOXYLATION MECHANISM. WHILE IBUPROFEN HAS WEAK ABSORPTION, IT HAS BEEN REPORTED AS A WEAK PHOTOSENSITISING AGENT.

DURING PREGNANCY

NSAIDS ARE NOT RECOMMENDED DURING PREGNANCY, PARTICULARLY DURING THE THIRD TRIMESTER. WHILE NSAIDS AS A CLASS IS NOT DIRECT TERATOGENS, THEY MAY CAUSE PREMATURE CLOSURE OF THE FETAL DUCTUS ARTERIOSUS AND RENAL ADRS IN THE FETUS. ADDITIONALLY, THEY ARE LINKED WITH PREMATURE BIRTH AND MISCARRIAGE. ASPIRIN, HOWEVER, IS USED TOGETHER WITH HEPARIN IN PREGNANT WOMEN WITH ANTIPHOSPHOLIPID ANTIBODIES. ADDITIONALLY, INDOMETHACIN IS USED IN PREGNANCY TO TREAT POLYHYDRAMNIOS BY REDUCING FETAL URINE PRODUCTION VIA INHIBITING FETAL RENAL BLOOD FLOW.

IN CONTRAST, PARACETAMOL (ACETAMINOPHEN) IS REGARDED AS BEING SAFE AND WELL-TOLERATED DURING PREGNANCY, BUT LEFFERS ET AL. RELEASED A STUDY IN 2010 INDICATING THAT THERE MAY BE ASSOCIATED MALE INFERTILITY IN THE UNBORN. DOSES SHOULD BE TAKEN AS PRESCRIBED, DUE TO RISK OF HEPATOTOXICITY WITH OVERDOSES.

IN FRANCE, THE COUNTRY'S HEALTH AGENCY CONTRAINDICATES THE USE OF NSAIDS, INCLUDING ASPIRIN, AFTER THE SIXTH MONTH OF PREGNANCY.

ALLERGY/ALLERGY-LIKE HYPERSENSITIVITY REACTIONS

A VARIETY OF ALLERGIC OR ALLERGIC-LIKE NSAID HYPERSENSITIVITY REACTIONS FOLLOW THE INGESTION OF NSAIDS. THESE HYPERSENSITIVITY REACTIONS DIFFER FROM THE OTHER ADVERSE REACTIONS LISTED HERE WHICH ARE TOXICITY REACTIONS, I.E. UNWANTED REACTIONS THAT RESULT FROM THE PHARMACOLOGICAL ACTION OF A DRUG, ARE DOSE-RELATED, AND CAN OCCUR IN ANY TREATED INDIVIDUAL; HYPERSENSITIVITY REACTIONS ARE IDIOSYNCRATIC REACTIONS TO A DRUG. SOME

NSAID HYPERSENSITIVITY REACTIONS ARE TRULY ALLERGIC IN ORIGIN:

1) REPETITIVE IGE-MEDIATED URTICARIAL SKIN ERUPTIONS, ANGIOEDEMA, AND ANAPHYLAXIS FOLLOWING IMMEDIATELY TO HOURS AFTER INGESTING ONE STRUCTURAL TYPE OF NSAID BUT NOT AFTER INGESTING STRUCTURALLY UNRELATED NSAIDS;

AND 2)COMPARATIVELY MILD TO MODERATELY SEVERE T CELL-MEDIATED DELAYED ONSET (USUALLY MORE THAN 24 HOUR), SKIN REACTIONS SUCH AS MACULOPAPULAR RASH, FIXED DRUG ERUPTIONS, PHOTOSENSITIVITY REACTIONS, DELAYED URTICARIA, AND CONTACT DERMATITIS;

OR 3) FAR MORE SEVERE AND POTENTIALLY LIFE-THREATENING T-CELL MEDIATED DELAYED SYSTEMIC REACTIONS SUCH AS THE DRESS SYNDROME, ACUTE GENERALIZED EXANTHEMATOUS PUSTULOSIS, THE STEVENS-JOHNSON SYNDROME, AND TOXIC EPIDERMAL NECROLYSIS. OTHER NSAID HYPERSENSITIVITY REACTIONS ARE ALLERGY-LIKE SYMPTOMS BUT DO NOT INVOLVE TRUE ALLERGIC MECHANISMS; RATHER, THEY APPEAR DUE TO THE ABILITY OF NSAIDS TO ALTER THE METABOLISM OF ARACHIDONIC ACID IN FAVOR OF FORMING METABOLITES THAT PROMOTE ALLERGIC SYMPTOMS. AFFLICTED INDIVIDUALS MAY BE ABNORMALLY SENSITIVE TO THESE PROVOCATIVE METABOLITES AND/OR OVERPRODUCE THEM AND TYPICALLY ARE SUSCEPTIBLE TO A WIDE RANGE OF STRUCTURALLY DISSIMILAR NSAIDS, PARTICULARLY THOSE THAT INHIBIT COX1. SYMPTOMS, WHICH DEVELOP IMMEDIATELY TO HOURS AFTER INGESTING ANY OF VARIOUS NSAIDS THAT INHIBIT COX-1, ARE:

1)EXACERBATIONS OF ASTHMATIC AND RHINITIS (SEE ASPIRIN-INDUCED ASTHMA) SYMPTOMS IN INDIVIDUALS WITH A HISTORY OF ASTHMA OR RHINITIS AND

2) EXACERBATION OR FIRST-TIME DEVELOPMENT OF WHEELS AND/OR ANGIOEDEMA IN INDIVIDUALS WITH OR WITHOUT A HISTORY OF CHRONIC URTICARIAL LESIONS OR ANGIOEDEMA.

Other

COMMON ADVERSE DRUG REACTIONS (ADR), OTHER THAN LISTED ABOVE, INCLUDE RAISED LIVER ENZYMES, HEADACHE, DIZZINESS. UNCOMMON ADRS INCLUDE HYPERKALAEMIA, CONFUSION,

BRONCHOSPASM, RASH. RAPID AND SEVERE SWELLING OF THE FACE AND/OR BODY. IBUPROFEN MAY ALSO RARELY CAUSE IRRITABLE BOWEL SYNDROME SYMPTOMS. NSAIDS ARE ALSO IMPLICATED IN SOME CASES OF STEVENS-JOHNSON SYNDROME. MOST NSAIDS PENETRATE POORLY INTO THE CENTRAL NERVOUS SYSTEM (CNS). HOWEVER, THE COX ENZYMES ARE EXPRESSED CONSTITUTIVELY IN SOME AREAS OF THE CNS, MEANING THAT EVEN LIMITED PENETRATION MAY CAUSE ADVERSE EFFECTS SUCH AS SOMNOLENCE AND DIZZINESS. IN VERY RARE CASES, IBUPROFEN CAN CAUSE ASEPTIC MENINGITIS. AS WITH OTHER DRUGS, ALLERGIES TO NSAIDS MIGHT EXIST. WHILE MANY ALLERGIES ARE SPECIFIC TO ONE NSAID, UP TO 1 IN 5 PEOPLE MAY HAVE UNPREDICTABLE CROSS-REACTIVE ALLERGIC RESPONSES TO OTHER NSAIDS AS WELL.

DRUG INTERACTIONS

NSAIDS REDUCE RENAL BLOOD FLOW AND THEREBY DECREASE THE EFFICACY OF DIURETICS, AND INHIBIT THE ELIMINATION OF LITHIUM AND METHOTREXATE. NSAIDS CAUSE HYPOCOAGULABILITY, WHICH MAY BE SERIOUS WHEN COMBINED WITH OTHER DRUGS THAT ALSO DECREASE BLOOD CLOTTING, SUCH AS WARFARIN. NSAIDS MAY AGGRAVATE HYPERTENSION (HIGH BLOOD PRESSURE) AND THEREBY ANTAGONIZE THE EFFECT OF ANTIHYPERTENSIVES, SUCH AS ACE INHIBITORS. NSAIDS MAY INTERFERE AND REDUCE EFFICIENCY OF SSRI ANTIDEPRESSANTS. VARIOUS WIDELY USED NONSTEROIDAL ANTI-INFLAMMATORY DRUGS (NSAIDS) ENHANCE ENDOCANNABINOID SIGNALING BY BLOCKING THE ANANDAMIDE-DEGRADING MEMBRANE ENZYME FATTY ACID AMIDE HYDROLASE (FAAH).

How's that for a warning label? Did it have enough side effects for you? Think you might need more meds after taking this one? That label was 4094 words long. How many of those did you read? How do you know what you're doing to your body if you don't know what you're putting into it? Do you think it a coincidence that Monsanto started their GMO seed about the same time that glycation started being researched? Since much of this kind of research is funded by the industry it affects, I wouldn't doubt that Monsanto had a hand in this research. This would allow them to immediately file these studies on glycation so that doctors and other scientists couldn't find them to review. It would also allow them to genetically modify their food to make it more fattening by allowing it to stand up to glyphosate herbicide. Yet each and every one of these 17,000+ studies has been vetted and examined by the NIH and PubMed. What I'd like to know is, why weren't warnings about glycation revealed then? Did Monsanto have anything to do with that?

The above list is the warning label for the adverse effects of Celebrex. Do you take Celebrex? Have you read the above warnings? Use of this drug can only lead to the use of more and more drugs. What do you think that would do for the profits for Monsanto and Pfizer? Do you still think this is a coincidence? From renal failure to the increased risk of myocardial infarction and stroke, this drug brings on more drug use, simply so people can get away from their pain. This pain is directly caused by the consumption of Monsanto's grains. To me, this is completely an unsustainable cycle. It's a cycle of hunger, dependence, disease, and death, leaving only people in pain. Where is the sense in keeping this addiction?

I propose that we tell Monsanto how we feel about this, not with our voices, but with our mouths in what we eat. All you have to do is quit eating grains. They're responsible for nearly all the pain you experience (with the exception of a few physical injuries).Grains and the glycation they bring, bring all inflammation that influences all diseases. Stop buying bread, crackers, cookies, anything that flour is used in, stop using it, forever. That's the only way you can start to free yourself from the addiction. You have to stop buying their junk food. Their comfort food is making you sick. It's making you sicker by the day.

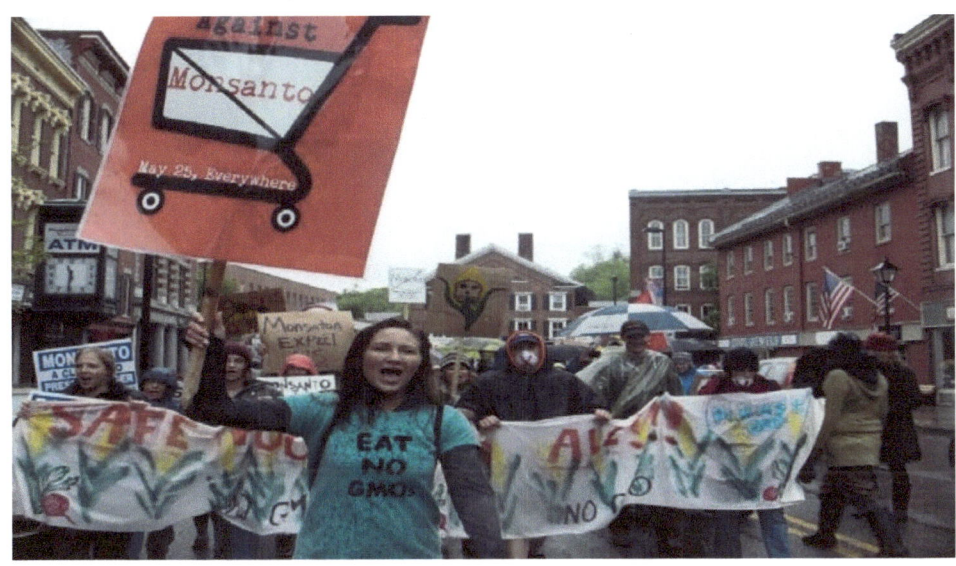

IT'S TIME TO TAKE OUR LIVES BACK!

PART III – REGULATION

WHOSE?

FDA's?

USDA's?

or

Monsanto's.

CHAPTER 8

FDA's Take on Gluten

Whose regulation, you ask? Who's not in this game. Who isn't even at first here. Only Monsanto is on any bases in this game. Monsanto controls all the bases in this game, from the FDA to the USDA to the CDC to probably the NIH, who houses and disseminates this information to the public as well. This to me is what's scary and why I won't buy into their ruse.

It would be nice if this was a problem with just the grain industry and Monsanto but it's not. It also involves the USDA and the FDA and what has influenced them to not issue warnings for this allergen and the effects it's having on the drug industry as well. The more I look at it, the more I see that it is a problem with overextending corporate entities intermingling their influence into regulatory agencies and offices to influence the agencies. Knowing the dealings that Monsanto has had in the past with competitors, regulatory agencies and offices, and their own judicial problems, it's not hard to fathom at all, the involvement they would have, in the non-disclosure of these studies. It's actually easy to see their involvement as being the same as the sugar industries', as they covered-up the studies showing their food as being this dangerous. They didn't just cover up the studies condemning glucose; they initiated reports themselves that showed glucose was healthy. That is a complete falsehood from the truth of what glucose does. What glucose does is the same thing that grains do, except that grains do it worse to you than the sugar does, because of the gliadin in the gluten that's in most grains.

Gluten does the same thing as sugar. Why won't the FDA recognize that? They have all the studies that point to it. Don't they read them?

The following is an excerpt from an FDA study on Gluten as an allergen (1 of 173 studies).

The Food Allergen Labeling and Consumer **Protection Act (FALCPA) of 2004**

FALCPA is an amendment to the Federal Food, Drug, and Cosmetic Act and requires that the label of a food that contains an ingredient that is or contains protein from a "major food allergen" declare the presence of the allergen in the manner described by the law.

Gluten

21. Why is there a concern about gluten?

Gluten describes a group of proteins found in certain grains (wheat, barley, and rye.) It is of concern because people with celiac disease cannot tolerate it. Celiac disease (also known as celiac sprue) is a chronic digestive disease that damages the small intestine and interferes with absorption of nutrients from food. Recent findings estimate that 2 million people in the U.S. have celiac disease or about 1 in 133 people.

22. What does FALCPA require with regard to gluten?

FALCPA requires FDA to issue a proposed rule that will define and permit the voluntary use of the term "gluten-free" on the labeling of foods by August 2006 and a final rule no later than August 2008.

23. What has FDA done in response to the FALCPA mandate?

FDA held a public meeting in August 2005 to obtain expert comment and consultation from stakeholders to help FDA develop a regulation to define and permit the voluntary use on food labeling of the term "gluten-free" (Public Meeting On Gluten-Free Food Labelling). The meeting focused on food manufacturing, analytical methods, and consumer issues related to reduced levels of gluten in food.

FDA's *gluten-free definition* is that the food contains less than 20 ppm of gluten.

They consider wheat and gluten as undeclared allergens yet they refuse to acknowledge its allergenic properties to the extent that they won't require a warning label for it. Yet they know what damage it does. This is evidenced by the reports listed in chapter 4. All they require is a mention of wheat in the ingredients and nothing more. That is their warning.

Their negligence in regards to our health in this manner is unconscionable. I can only assume that they've been influenced by the other side of the industry that provides crop seed for the farmers that grow the food that the FDA approves for us to eat. The other side of this industry, owned by the same corporations, is the pharmaceutical industry. They provide us with all of the drugs that we take to fight the disease caused by the food provided their sister crop seed industry.

What I wonder is, what does the FDA consider stakeholders? Are they the corporate entities who have an interest in proliferating wheat and gluten?

Since we now know that this happened with sugar, why wouldn't the same thing happen with gluten? We know that gluten breaks down into nothing more than glucose, I can see where the same situation would exist today, that existed 50 -60 years ago. In fact, I believe it's an ongoing problem that won't be resolved until the consumer does something about it.

Just like in the tobacco industry, "selling a product that is already sold for them as it's addictive", the same mantra is heard in the grain industry concerning their gluten. "How can people refuse to buy our products? They're addictive so people will want them more and more of them. The beauty of this addiction is that it feeds the other side of the same industry, the pharmaceutical industry.

I salute the FDA for monitoring products claiming to be gluten-free yet have more than a trace of gluten in them, such as the *Investigation* into General Mills for selling Cheerio's that had more than the allowed limit of 20 ppm of gluten. Yet knowing what damage gluten does to the body, I have to wonder why do they still allow it to be marketed without any warnings? The tobacco companies can't market their products without warnings. Why is the food industry allowed to? The evidence lies within the vaults of the NIH's PubMed, showing all the damage it does. Why do they ignore that evidence? I think it has to do with not enough funds or people to look over these studies. There is – after all – over 11,685 studies done on the glycation which is caused by the digestion of gluten to introduce glucose into your blood. That was the last count a couple days ago. Today I don't know how many research studies have been added. When I first checked last week, there were 11,667. This is something that is that important, yet the neither the FDA nor the USDA says anything about its dangers.

What dangers, you say? The evidence lies in the excerpts below, from 10 of their 173 studies on gluten;

1. *"GLUTEN IS THE PROTEIN THAT NATURALLY OCCURS IN WHEAT, RYE, BARLEY, AND CROSSBREEDS OF THESE GRAINS. MOST PEOPLE CAN EAT GLUTEN, BUT IN PEOPLE WITH CELIAC DISEASE, GLUTEN INTAKE GRADUALLY DAMAGES THE INTESTINES, PREVENTS THE ABSORPTION OF VITAMINS AND MINERALS, AND CAN LEAD TO OTHER HEALTH PROBLEMS. SYMPTOMS CAN INCLUDE DIARRHEA, FATIGUE, HEADACHES, ABDOMINAL PAIN, BRAIN FOG, RASHES, NAUSEA, VOMITING, AND OTHER REACTIONS."*
2. *"PEOPLE WHO HAVE AN ALLERGY TO WHEAT RUN THE RISK OF SERIOUS OR LIFE-THREATENING ALLERGIC REACTION IF THEY EAT WHEAT. SYMPTOMS MAY INCLUDE SWELLING, ITCHING OR IRRITATION OF MOUTH OR THROAT, DIFFICULTY BREATHING, NASAL CONGESTION, ITCHY OR WATERY EYES, RASH OR HIVES, HEADACHES, NAUSEA, VOMITING, CRAMPS, DIARRHEA, OR ANAPHYLAXIS, A POTENTIALLY LIFE-THREATENING REACTION."*

What I can't understand, with this kind of disruption of bodily functions, why doesn't this require a warning like cigarettes? It's clearly killed more people.

3. *"UNLIKE FOOD ALLERGIES, CLINICAL SIGNS AND SYMPTOMS DO NOT APPEAR TO BE RELIABLE MARKERS OF DISEASE ACTIVITY BECAUSE MANY INDIVIDUALS AFFECTED WITH CELIAC DISEASE MAY BE ENTIRELY ASYMPTOMATIC.* This tells me that a lot more people suffer from the disease than what has been diagnosed. *FURTHERMORE, ALTHOUGH BIOMARKERS OF GENETIC SUSCEPTIBILITY (E.G., PRESENCE OF DQ2 AND/OR DQ8 HLA ALLELES) AND GLUTEN EXPOSURE [E.G., ANTIBODIES FOR GLIADIN (AGA), ENDOMYSIAL (EMA), AND TISSUE TRANSGLUTAMINASE (TTG)] HAVE BEEN DEFINED FOR USE IN NONINVASIVE DIAGNOSIS OF INDIVIDUALS WITH CELIAC DISEASE, THESE BIOMARKERS HAVE NOT BEEN SHOWN TO CORRELATE WITH DISEASE SEVERITY NOR TO BE USEFUL IN ASSESSING DAILY RESPONSES TO GLUTEN EXPOSURES. RATHER, EVIDENCE OF INTESTINAL MUCOSAL INFLAMMATION IS THE GOLD STANDARD BIOMARKER FOR DIAGNOSIS OF CELIAC DISEASE AND FOR ASSESSMENT OF DISEASE SEVERITY. INTESTINAL MUCOSAL INFLAMMATION MAY OCCUR LONG BEFORE THE DEVELOPMENT OF CLINICAL SIGNS OR A RISE IN ANTIBODY TITERS FOLLOWING A GLUTEN CHALLENGE. INTESTINAL INFLAMMATION IS ASSESSED BY INTESTINAL BIOPSY, WHICH IS AN INVASIVE PROCEDURE, ASSOCIATED WITH FALSE NEGATIVES (DUE TO SAMPLING ERROR), AND IS IMPRACTICAL FOR FREQUENT MONITORING OF DISEASE ACTIVITY OR SEVERITY." REVISED THRESHOLD REPORT PAGE 58 OF 108*

4. *"UNPUBLISHED DATA DESCRIBED IN MONERET-VAUTRIN AND KANNY (2004) SHOW THAT 83% OF WHEAT ALLERGIC CHILDREN REACTED TO LESS THAN 2 G OF WHEAT FLOUR WHILE ONLY 18% OF WHEAT ALLERGIC ADULTS responded at this level. Unpublished data described in Moneret Vautrin (2004) on wheat flour CHALLENGES USING 32 CHILDREN AND 32 ADULTS WITH WHEAT ALLERGY, REPORTED A LOAEL OF ≤ 1.8 MG PROTEIN FOR ALLERGIC CHILDREN (THE LOWEST TESTED DOSE) AND 52.8 MG PROTEIN FOR ALLERGIC ADULTS. SCIBILIA ET AL. (2006) REPORTED THAT 2 OF 13 RESPONDERS REACTED TO THE LOWEST DOSE OF WHEAT FLOUR TESTED (100 MG OF A MIX OF BREAD AND DURUM FLOUR, APPROXIMATELY 15 MG PROTEIN) IN DBPCFCS. IN TOTAL, 31% OF THE PATIENTS WHO REACTED DID SO TO CHALLENGE DOSES LESS THAN OR EQUAL TO 240 MG OF WHEAT PROTEIN." APPROACHES TO ESTABLISH THRESHOLDS FOR MAJOR FOOD ALLERGENS* My question is how many people eat this amount? Most people eat around 150mg of wheat products in a day, not enough to express symptoms of celiac disease, but enough to do unnoticed damage.

5. *"THE FOODS OF CONCERN FOR INDIVIDUALS WITH, OR SUSCEPTIBLE TO, CELIAC DISEASE ARE THE CEREAL GRAINS*

THAT CONTAIN THE STORAGE PROTEINS PROLAMIN AND GLUTELIN (COMMONLY REFERRED TO AS GLUTENS IN WHEAT), INCLUDING ALL VARIETIES OF WHEAT (E.G., DURUM, SPELT, KAMUT), BARLEY (WHERE THE STORAGE PROTEINS ARE CALLED HORDES), RYE (WHERE THE STORAGE PROTEINS ARE CALLED SECALINS), AND THEIR CROSS-BRED HYBRIDS (SUCH AS TRITICALE). THE PROPORTION OF INDIVIDUALS WITH CELIAC DISEASE THAT ARE ALSO SENSITIVE TO THE STORAGE PROTEINS IN OATS (AVENINS) HAS NOT BEEN DETERMINED BUT IS LIKELY TO BE LESS THAN 1% (KELLY, 2005)."

6. *"THE CLINICAL MANIFESTATIONS OF CELIAC DISEASE ARE HIGHLY VARIABLE IN CHARACTER AND SEVERITY. THE REASONS FOR THIS DIVERSITY ARE UNKNOWN BUT MAY DEPEND ON THE AGE AND IMMUNOLOGICAL STATUS OF THE INDIVIDUAL, THE AMOUNT, DURATION, OR TIMING OF EXPOSURE TO GLUTEN, AND THE SPECIFIC AREA AND EXTENT OF THE GASTROINTESTINAL TRACT INVOLVED BY DISEASE (DEWAR ET AL., 2004). THESE CLINICAL MANIFESTATIONS CAN BE DIVIDED INTO GASTROINTESTINAL, OR "CLASSIC," AND NON-GASTROINTESTINAL MANIFESTATIONS. GASTROINTESTINAL MANIFESTATIONS USUALLY PRESENT IN CHILDREN 4 TO 24 MONTHS OLD AND INCLUDE ABDOMINAL PAIN AND CRAMPING, BLOATING, RECURRENT OR CHRONIC DIARRHEA IN ASSOCIATION WITH WEIGHT LOSS, POOR GROWTH, NUTRIENT DEFICIENCY, AND (IN RARE CASES) A LIFE-THREATENING METABOLIC EMERGENCY TERMED CELIAC CRISIS, CHARACTERIZED BY HYPOKALEMIA AND ACIDOSIS SECONDARY TO PROFUSE DIARRHEA (FARRELL AND KELLY, 2002; BARANWAL ET AL., 2003). NON-GASTROINTESTINAL MANIFESTATIONS ARE MORE INSIDIOUS AND HIGHLY VARIABLE AND ARE THE COMMON PRESENTING SIGNS IN OLDER CHILDREN AND ADULTS. THESE MANIFESTATIONS ARE FREQUENTLY THE RESULT OF LONG-TERM NUTRIENT MALABSORPTION, INCLUDING IRON DEFICIENCY ANEMIA, SHORT STATURE, DELAYED PUBERTY, INFERTILITY, AND OSTEOPOROSIS OR OSTEOPENIA (FASANO, 2003). IN CHILDREN, PROGRESSIVE MALABSORPTION OF NUTRIENTS MAY LEAD TO GROWTH, DEVELOPMENTAL, OR NEUROLOGICAL DELAYS (CATASSI AND FASANO, 2004). EXTRA-INTESTINAL MANIFESTATIONS SUCH AS DERMATITIS HERPETIFORMIS, HEPATITIS, PERIPHERAL NEUROPATHY, ATAXIA, AND EPILEPSY HAVE ALSO BEEN ASSOCIATED WITH CELIAC DISEASE (FASANO AND CATASSI, 2001). INDIVIDUALS WITH UNTREATED CELIAC DISEASE ARE ALSO AT INCREASED RISK FOR POTENTIALLY SERIOUS MEDICAL CONDITIONS, SUCH AS OTHER AUTOIMMUNE DISEASES (E.G., TYPE I DIABETES MELLITUS) AND INTESTINAL CANCERS ASSOCIATED WITH HIGH MORTALITY (FARRELL AND KELLY, 2002; PETERS ET AL., 2003; CATASSI ET AL., 2002). FOR EXAMPLE, INDIVIDUALS WITH CELIAC DISEASE HAVE AN 80-FOLD GREATER RISK OF DEVELOPING ADENOCARCINOMA OF THE SMALL INTESTINE, A GREATER THAN TWO-FOLD INCREASED RISK*

FOR INTESTINAL OR EXTRA INTESTINAL LYMPHOMAS (GREEN AND JABRI, 2003) AND A 20-FOLD GREATER RISK OF DEVELOPING ENTEROPATHY-ASSOCIATED T CELL LYMPHOMA (EATL) (CATASSI ET AL.,"

7. *"THERE IS NO STANDARD PROTOCOL FOR GLUTEN CHALLENGES, AND CHALLENGE STUDIES HAVE VARIED GREATLY IN AMOUNT AND DURATION OF GLUTEN EXPOSURE. ALTHOUGH SOME STUDIES HAVE BEEN DESIGNED TO DETERMINE THE ACUTE EFFECTS (I.E., AFTER 4 HOURS) OF EXPOSURE TO GLUTEN (STURGESS AL., 1994; CICLITIRAET AL., 1984), MOST CHALLENGES CONSIST OF AN OPEN CHALLENGE TO A FIXED OR INCREMENTAL DOSE OF DAILY GLUTEN OVER A MINIMUM PERIOD OF 4 WEEKS. MANY CHALLENGE STUDIES USE A HIGH EXPOSURE (≥ 10 G/DAY) TO GLUTEN BECAUSE THIS IS BELIEVED TO SHORTEN TIME TO DISEASE CONFIRMATION OR RELAPSE AND, THEREFORE, TO MINIMIZE DISCOMFORT TO SUBJECTS (ROLLES AND MCNEISH, 1976). HOWEVER, SOME STUDIES HAVE SHOWN THAT LOW DAILY EXPOSURES TO GLUTEN ALSO CAN ELICIT A DISEASE RESPONSE (CATASSI ET AL., 1993; LAURIN ET AL., 2002; HAMILTON AND MCNEILL, 1972)."*

8. *"AT THIS TIME THERE IS NO CORRELATIVE INFORMATION ON THE EFFICACY OF USING THESE TESTS TO PREDICT OR HELP PREVENT ADVERSE EFFECTS IN INDIVIDUALS WITH CELIAC DISEASE."*

9. *"ALTHOUGH GLUTEN-FREE DIETS ARE CONSIDERED THE ONLY EFFECTIVE TREATMENT FOR INDIVIDUALS WITH CELIAC DISEASE, IT HAS BEEN RECOGNIZED THAT IT IS DIFFICULT, IF NOT IMPOSSIBLE, TO MAINTAIN A DIET THAT IS COMPLETELY DEVOID OF GLUTEN (COLLINET AL., 2004). THEREFORE, SEVERAL ATTEMPTS HAVE BEEN MADE TO DEFINE GLUTEN-FREE IN REGULATORY CONTEXTS. EFFORTS BY THE CODEX ALIMENTARIUS TO DEFINE AN INTERNATIONAL STANDARD FOR "GLUTEN-FREE" LABELING DATE BACK TO 1981. AT THAT TIME, DUE TO THE LACK OF SENSITIVE, SPECIFIC ANALYTICAL METHODS, A THRESHOLD VALUE OF 0.05 G NITROGEN PER 100 G DRY MATTER WAS SET FOR WHEAT STARCH, ON THE ASSUMPTION THAT WHEAT PROTEIN WOULD BE THE ONLY SOURCE OF NITROGEN IN STARCH (CODEX STANDARD 118-1981). THE CODEX COMMITTEE ON NUTRITION AND FOODS FOR SPECIAL DIETARY USES IS DEVELOPING A REVISED STANDARD. THE CURRENT DRAFT PROPOSAL WOULD DEFINE THREE CATEGORIES OF GLUTEN-FREE FOODS: PROCESSED FOODS THAT ARE NATURALLY "GLUTEN-FREE" (≤ 20 PPM OF GLUTEN), PRODUCTS THAT HAD BEEN RENDERED "GLUTEN-FREE" BY PROCESSING (≤ 200 PPM), AND ANY MIXTURE OF THE TWO (≤ 200 PPM). THE AUSTRALIA NEW ZEALAND FOOD AGENCY (ANZFA) DEFINES GLUTEN TO MEAN "THE MAIN PROTEIN IN WHEAT, RYE, OATS, BARLEY, TRITICALE AND SPELT RELEVANT TO THE MEDICAL CONDITIONS, COELIAC DISEASE, AND DERMATITIS*

HEPETIFORMIS." ANZFA RECOGNIZES TWO CLASSES OF FOODS, GLUTEN-FREE FOODS (" ...NO DETECTABLE GLUTEN") AND LOW-GLUTEN FOODS (" ...NO MORE THAN 20 MG GLUTEN PER 100 GM OF THE FOOD") (ANZFA FOOD CODE STANDARD 1.2.8). THE CANADIAN STANDARD FOR "GLUTEN-FREE" IS MORE GENERAL, SIMPLY STATING THAT "NO PERSON SHALL LABEL, PACKAGE, SELL OR ADVERTISE A FOOD IN A MANNER LIKELY TO CREATE AN IMPRESSION THAT IT IS A "GLUTEN-FREE" FOOD UNLESS THE FOOD DOES NOT CONTAIN WHEAT, INCLUDING SPELT AND KAMUT, OR OATS, BARLEY, RYE, TRITICALE OR ANY PART THEREOF" (CANADIAN FOOD AND DRUGS ACT REGULATION B.24.018)." APPROACHES TO ESTABLISH THRESHOLDS FOR MAJOR FOOD ALLERGENS AND FOR GLUTEN IN FOOD. III, IV, V.

Now that you know what grains this involves you can get an idea of what not to eat.

10. *"LIKE FOOD ALLERGIES, CELIAC DISEASE AFFECTS ONLY A SMALL PROPORTION OF THE U.S. POPULATION (ESTIMATED AT 1%, 3.1 MILLION) (NIH, 2004). SUSCEPTIBILITY TO CELIAC DISEASE IS GENETICALLY DETERMINED AND IS LINKED TO THE PRESENCE OF THE DQ2 OR DQ8 HLA ALLELES. HOWEVER, CARRYING THESE ALLELES DOES NOT NECESSARILY LEAD TO CELIAC DISEASE. BOTH ACUTE AND CHRONIC MORBIDITY HAVE BEEN WELL DOCUMENTED FOR INDIVIDUALS WITH SYMPTOMATIC CELIAC DISEASE. A GLUTEN-FREE DIET HAS BEEN SHOWN TO GREATLY REDUCE THE RISK FOR CANCER AND OVERALL MORTALITY FOR THESE INDIVIDUALS. THE POTENTIAL BENEFIT OF A GLUTEN-FREE DIET HAS NOT BEEN ESTABLISHED FOR INDIVIDUALS WITH SILENT OR LATENT CELIAC DISEASE."*

I submit that this is a disease of a much grander scale, than what's reported, as far too often this disease goes completely unrecognized and thus undiagnosed. I hear complaints from many carboholics about many of the disorders at the top of this list. That tells me that they each have an allergic intolerance to gluten and they don't even know it. Because of its addictive nature, they'll never know it, unless they can give it up. The above paragraphs apply to those with celiac disease, yet I contend that everyone experiences some of the above reactions to some degree. This happens even more so if you consume more of their products. I thought

I could eat this food for 58 years until I learned that I had allergies to it. Now I know that I have numerous allergic intolerances to this food. They present themselves every time I try to eat it again.

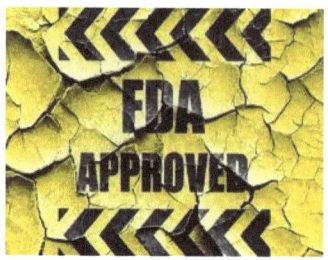

My guess is that 95% of the population is exactly the same as I am, allergic to the protein in gluten. I contend that the obesity and diabetes rates that exist today confirm this. The death rates of all the diseases caused by glycation prove it. That forces me to ask, with all the evidence available in your archives FDA, why doesn't this food require a warning?

They require other carcinogens to display warnings. Why not this one? This food is not only carcinogenic; it's atherosclerotic and inflammatory. What more could you want in a poison?

This is what the FDA claims they're concerned about;

"IN 21 CODE OF FEDERAL REGULATIONS (CFR) PART 117 (PART 117), WE HAVE ESTABLISHED OUR REGULATION ENTITLED "CURRENT GOOD MANUFACTURING PRACTICE, HAZARD ANALYSIS, AND RISK-BASED PREVENTIVE CONTROLS FOR HUMAN FOOD." WE PUBLISHED THE FINAL RULE ESTABLISHING PART 117 IN THE FEDERAL REGISTER OF SEPTEMBER 17, 2015 (80 FR 55908). PART 117 ESTABLISHES REQUIREMENTS FOR CURRENT GOOD MANUFACTURING PRACTICE FOR HUMAN FOOD (CGMPS), FOR HAZARD ANALYSIS AND RISK-BASED PREVENTIVE CONTROLS FOR HUMAN FOOD (PCHF), AND RELATED REQUIREMENTS."

After reviewing over half of the documents available and an examination of all the titles of the documents, I see nothing that bans the inclusion of any of these dangerous foods in our food products made for public consumption (processed foods, including bread). It seems their interest lies only in compliance with the labeling of the product. They want to make sure that a package that's sold as gluten-free has to have less than 20ppm gluten in the product.

They don't even feel that it's important enough to warn you that a product contains gluten, and they don't feel it important enough to warn you of the dangers of gluten on the package like they do with the dangers of cigarettes. They recognize the danger of tobacco, why can't they recognize the dangers of gluten and wheat? It seems that they're content with the warning you how much a product is gluten-free, but not how much gluten it has in it as if it does no harm at all. C'MON MAN. I have access to the same studies they have. They're all located at PUBMED.COM and they all explain the dangers this food presents. If I can learn about what this food does, they have to know. Why are they so willing to ignore it? Why are they so willing to treat this food as though there's nothing wrong with it?

The first page of studies I opened brought me to this study, the twelfth study out of 1797 studies on the list and reveals the dangers of just breathing the dust from these cereal grains. The grain induced asthma which affects those who work in the various fields in the grain industry, as stated by the Allergy, Asthma & Immunology Research:

"ASTHMA CAUSED BY ALLERGY TO PROTEINS FROM CEREAL GRAINS IS ONE OF THE MOST COMMON TYPES OF OCCUPATIONAL ASTHMA (OA) AND ITS PREVALENCE DOES NOT SEEM TO BE DECLINING. THE MAIN PROFESSIONS AFFECTED ARE: BAKERS, CONFECTIONERS, PASTRY FACTORY WORKERS, MILLERS, FARMERS, AND CEREAL HANDLERS. ALTHOUGH WHEAT IS THE MOST COMMONLY INVOLVED CEREAL, OTHER GRAINS (E.G. RYE, BARLEY, RICE) ALSO PLAY A ROLE. IN ADDITION, FLOUR FROM OTHER SOURCES (E.G. SOYA, LUPIN), PESTS, AND SEVERAL FLOUR ADDITIVES USED IN THE BAKING INDUSTRY TO IMPROVE FERMENTATION AND ELASTICITY OF THE DOUGH, AS WELL AS TO IMPROVE STORAGE OF THE BREAD, MAY ALSO GIVE RISE TO IGE-MEDIATED ALLERGY." "THIS DISORDER HAS BEEN CLASSICALLY CONSIDERED A FORM OF ALLERGIC ASTHMA MEDIATED BY IGE ANTIBODIES SPECIFIC TO CEREAL FLOUR ANTIGENS, MAINLY WHEAT, RYE, AND BARLEY,"

In the tenth study on the list published, in July 2009, it's been found that the globulins in wheat can cause type1 diabetes. T1D is an autoimmune disorder that was thought to have no cause. At least, all the studies I've looked at didn't reveal this. According to *BioMed Central*;

"TAKEN TOGETHER, THE RESULTS INDICATE THAT A DIVERSE GROUP OF GLOBULINS EXISTS IN WHEAT, SOME OF WHICH COULD BE ASSOCIATED WITH THE PATHOGENESIS OF T1D IN SOME SUSCEPTIBLE INDIVIDUALS. THESE DATA EXPAND OUR KNOWLEDGE OF SPECIFIC WHEAT GLOBULINS AND WILL ENABLE FURTHER ELUCIDATION OF THEIR ROLE IN WHEAT BIOLOGY AND HUMAN HEALTH.

I have read elsewhere that it might be thought that an allergen might trigger an autoimmune response that shuts down the hormones that trigger insulin manufacture in the pancreas. It appears that this is that finding. Wheat can be responsible for type 1 diabetes. Have you seen any warnings for that? I haven't. Have any been issued? I haven't seen them. Why haven't they been issued? How many parents have fed their kids bread to find out that their children are diabetic because of this auto-immune disorder? Why is bread still considered by so many to be a necessity of life? It doesn't appear so. It appears more likely to be a destroyer of life.

We can end this. We can change our diet.

This is what I'm concerned about;

47,397 deaths every day from CVDs

THE ATHEROSCLEROTIC EFFECT

47,397 people died each day, worldwide, from cardiovascular disease in 2013. That breaks down to over 1800 Americans that died every day from cardiovascular disease in 2013. That's about 79 people every hour. That's 17.3 million annually, worldwide. That was up from 12.3 million (25.8%) in 1990. According to Wikipedia;

"CORONARY ARTERY DISEASE AND STROKE ACCOUNT FOR 80% OF CVD DEATHS IN MALES AND 75% OF CVD DEATHS IN FEMALES. MOST CARDIOVASCULAR DISEASE AFFECTS OLDER ADULTS. IN THE UNITED STATES 11% OF PEOPLE BETWEEN 20 AND 40 HAVE CVD, WHILE 37% BETWEEN 40 AND 60, 71% OF PEOPLE BETWEEN 60 AND 80, AND 85% OF PEOPLE OVER 80 HAVE CVD. THE AVERAGE AGE OF DEATH FROM CORONARY ARTERY DISEASE IN THE DEVELOPED WORLD IS AROUND 80 WHILE IT IS AROUND 68 IN THE DEVELOPING WORLD."

This rate is increasing each year by an ever-increasing rate, outpacing itself every year. This statement proves how slow this damage of glycation manifests. But it does manifest every time you eat anything that breaks down into glucose. And that includes all carbs, all sugars.

THE CARCINOGENIC EFFECT

According to the NCBI's PubMed;
A total of 1,658,370 new cancer cases and 589,430 cancer deaths are projected to occur in the United States in 2015.

1614 Americans die every day from cancer, in the US alone, due to ECC. That's 67 people every hour who die from cancer in the US alone. My mother was one of them. That's why I wrote this book. I know I'm not alone in the way I feel about the despair of cancer and number of lives it ruins. The changes that have to be made to correct this dilemma that our food industry has inflicted upon us have to be made with a concerted effort by everyone involved. Otherwise, the health of our society will never recover.
Consumers should stop buying this food so that the manufacturers and growers will start growing and manufacturing something else more nutritious.

THE INFLAMMATORY EFFECT

In 2015, there were approximately 48 million people worldwide with the AD. In 2010, dementia resulted in about 486,000 deaths, according to Wikipedia. That's 19,440 Americans every year. That's 53 people every day that this disease takes and it won't stop until you stop the glycation. The only way you can stop the glycation is to take away the glucose that triggers it. This is curable. It's going to require that everyone conquer their own addiction. That means that the food industry has to stop starting the addiction by keeping it out of all baby food. Their refusal to do so is your proof of where it starts. If other natural sweeteners (that aren't addictive) were put in baby food instead of sugar, It might stop the start of the addiction. But sugar is still considered safe to eat, by USDA and FDA standards.

How many people do you know who aren't affected by arthritis? I only know of a few who claim that they aren't. Arthritis is the widest spread manifestations of glycation. This is due to the fact that inflammation exists in the blood and it affects every bone and organ that your blood flows through. Because of this, the arthritis is always the first to be felt. The other manifestations usually aren't felt until it is too late. That's the manifestations of atherosclerosis and cancer and Alzheimer's disease. By the time you feel those, you're already deep into the drug cycle, and that's a cycle that ends only in death or abstinence.

Probably the first of these inflammatory manifestations to fully hit you is IBF or a condition preceding Irritable Bowel Syndrome as this is a major disorder that can be attributed directly to inflammation as evidenced by this report submitted Dec 16 last year;

BACKGROUND:
Irritable bowel syndrome (IBS) and inflammatory bowel disease (IBD) patients report similar gastrointestinal (GI) symptoms, yet comparisons of symptom severity between groups and with the general population (GP) are lacking.
The Overlap between Irritable Bowel Syndrome and Non-Celiac Gluten Sensitivity: A Clinical Dilemma
The spectrum of gluten-related disorders has widened in recent times and includes celiac disease, non-celiac gluten sensitivity, and wheat allergy. The complex of symptoms associated with these diseases, such as diarrhea, constipation or abdominal pain may overlap for the gluten-related diseases, and furthermore, they can be similar to those caused by various other intestinal diseases, such as irritable bowel syndrome (IBS). The mechanisms underlying symptom generation are diverse for all these diseases. Some patients with celiac disease may remain asymptomatic or have only mild gastrointestinal symptoms and thus may qualify for the diagnosis of IBS in the general clinical practice. Similarly, the overlap of symptoms between IBS and non-celiac gluten sensitivity (NCGS) often creates a

dilemma for clinicians. While the treatment of NCGS is the exclusion of gluten from the diet, some, but not all, of the patients with IBS also improve on a gluten-free diet. Both IBS and NCGS are common in the general population and both can coexist with each other independently without necessarily sharing a common pathophysiological basis. Although the pathogenesis of NCGS is not well understood, it is likely to be heterogeneous with possible contributing factors such as low-grade intestinal inflammation, increased intestinal barrier function and changes in the intestinal microbiota. Innate immunity may also play a pivotal role. One possible inducer of innate immune response has recently been reported to be an amylase-trypsin inhibitor, a protein present in wheat endosperm and the source of flour, along with the gluten proteins.

The question I keep asking myself is why does this have to keep happening? Why hasn't the FDA warned us about the dangers of this food? They have access to all of the same reports that I do, yet they still refuse to acknowledge that this food is dangerous. Does their interest lie elsewhere? Is there corporate influence involved with this, like there was with sugar? This is sugar! So why are they still covering it up?

"The sugar industry actively took steps for years to influence public's perception of the nutritional value of their product, when they clearly knew of the dangers it posed. "Food companies have spent billions of dollars to cover up the link between sugar consumption and health problems. That's the conclusion of a new report from the Center for Science and Democracy at the Union of Concerned Scientists (UCS)."

According to *The Guardian*;

"SUGAR LOBBY PAID SCIENTISTS TO BLUR SUGAR'S ROLE IN HEART DISEASE" – REPORT

"New report highlights battle by the industry to counter sugar's negative health effects, and the cushy relationship between food companies and researchers". " Influential research that downplayed the role of sugar in heart disease in the 1960s was paid for by the sugar industry, according to a report released on Monday.

These actions are responsible for more deaths than all the world wars combined. Their actions have killed, hurt or harmed more than 500,000,000 people in the last 30 years alone. (At 17.3 million for heart disease alone, 500 million is a lowball estimate for death coming from cancer and dementia as well.) All total, the death rate for **ECC** is over 24,000,000 each year.

That's over 65,753 deaths each day, simply from excessive carbohydrate consumption. (Remember carbs = sugar.)

With backing from a sugar lobby, scientists promoted dietary fat as the cause of coronary heart disease instead of sugar, according to a historical document review published in JAMA Internal Medicine. This was criminal, yet nothing was done about it.

Though the review is nearly 50 years old, it showcases a decades-long battle by the sugar industry to persuade the public about the product's positive health effects, when it really has had none, ever. Why isn't this agency being held accountable? Maybe we should review who controls the agencies of the FDA and the USDA. (Knowing Monsanto, I wouldn't doubt the EPA also.)

The findings come from documents recently found by a researcher at the University of San Francisco, which show that scientists at the Sugar Research Foundation (SRF), known today as the Sugar Association, paid scientists to do a 1967 literature review that overlooked the role of sugar in heart disease. Wasn't that a clear case of bribery that should have been prosecuted?

SRF set an objective for the review, funded it and reviewed drafts before it was published in the New England Journal of Medicine, which did not require conflict of interest disclosure until 1984. The three Harvard scientists who wrote the review made what would be $50,000 in today's dollars from the review. Because of this bribery, over 500,000,000 have suffered from these diseases that sugar is responsible for. From diabetes to heart disease to dementia to cancer to arthritis (you should be familiar with the list by now).

Marion Nestle, nutrition, food studies and public health professor at New York University, said the food industry continues to influence nutrition science, in an editorial published alongside the JAMA report;
"TODAY, IT IS ALMOST IMPOSSIBLE TO KEEP UP WITH THE RANGE OF FOOD COMPANIES SPONSORING RESEARCH – FROM MAKERS OF THE MOST HIGHLY PROCESSED FOODS, DRINKS, AND SUPPLEMENTS TO PRODUCERS OF DAIRY FOODS, MEATS, FRUITS, AND NUTS – TYPICALLY YIELDING RESULTS FAVORABLE TO THE SPONSOR'S INTERESTS," NESTLE SAID. "FOOD COMPANY SPONSORSHIP, WHETHER OR NOT INTENTIONALLY MANIPULATIVE, UNDERMINES PUBLIC TRUST IN NUTRITION SCIENCE, CONTRIBUTES TO PUBLIC CONFUSION ABOUT WHAT TO EAT, AND COMPROMISES DIETARY GUIDELINES IN WAYS THAT ARE NOT IN THE BEST INTEREST OF PUBLIC HEALTH."

"THE CUSHY RELATIONSHIP BETWEEN FOOD COMPANIES AND RESEARCHER HAS BEEN CAPTURED IN RECENT INVESTIGATIONS BY THE ASSOCIATED PRESS AND NEW YORK TIMES. THE AP REVEALED IN JUNE THAT CANDY TRADE GROUPS WERE FUNDING RESEARCH INTO SWEETS. AND IN 2015, THE NEW YORK TIMES SHOWED HOW COCA-COLA HAS FUNDED MILLIONS IN RESEARCH TO DOWNPLAY THE LINK BETWEEN SUGARY BEVERAGES AND OBESITY."

The Sugar Association said in a statement that SRF *"should have exercised greater transparency" in its research, but also accused the study authors of having an "anti-sugar narrative".*

"We question this author's continued attempts to reframe historical occurrences to conveniently align with the currently trending anti-sugar narrative, particularly when the last several decades of research have concluded that sugar does not have a unique role in heart disease," the Sugar Association said. "Most concerning is the growing use of headline-baiting articles to trump quality scientific research – we're disappointed to see a journal of JAMA's stature being drawn into this trend."

The findings were based on documents found by Cristin Kearns, a postdoctoral fellow at UCSF, in library archives. The scientists and executives involved are no longer alive.

In recent years, the link between fat and heart disease has become a more contentious topic – a 2010 review of scientific studies of fat in the American Journal of Clinical Nutrition found that "there is no convincing evidence that saturated fat causes heart disease". The role of sugar in heart disease is still being debated."

Even according to Mother Jones;

"The industry's tactics—similar to those used by Big Tobacco in downplaying the adverse health effects of smoking—were explored by Gary Taubes and Cristin Kearns Couzens in the 2012 Mother Jones investigation "Big Sugar's Sweet Little Lies." But this latest report draws on some newly released documents submitted as evidence in a recent federal court case involving the two biggest players in the sweetener industry: the Sugar Association and the Corn Refiners Association (the trade group for manufacturers of high fructose corn syrup). "

When will it stop?
Until we let this industry know that we won't accept their definition of healthy food and stop buying their versions of it, you're going to be eating it until you

start buying their drugs. And you'll still keep eating it. Only when it becomes unprofitable will it be eliminated.

"Obesity and diabetes mellitus are often linked to cardiovascular disease, as are a history of chronic kidney disease and hypercholesterolemia. In fact, cardiovascular disease is the most life-threatening of the diabetic complications and diabetics are two- to four-fold more likely to die of cardiovascular-related causes than nondiabetics."

According to the World Heart Association;

"Up to 90% of cardiovascular disease may be preventable if established risk factors are avoided. " Their goal is 25 by 25. "25x25, achieving a 25% relative reduction in overall mortality from cardiovascular disease, cancer, diabetes or chronic respiratory disease by 2025. In September 2011, the United Nations held a High-Level Meeting in New York on the subject of CDs, including cardiovascular disease (CVD), cancers, diabetes and chronic respiratory diseases."

They're actively taking steps to lower the death rate of CVDs by recommending everyone to eat right, quit smoking, and exercise, all of which will lower this number one killer of people. Eating right, in my opinion, is by far the best way to combat CVD, diabetes, obesity, hypertension, high cholesterol (which is really a problem of unbalanced cholesterol), arthritis and worst of all, dementia and Alzheimer disease.

In all of my research, I can't find anything that says to limit the use of bread and starchy carbohydrates made from grains. Yet all research I've looked at from PubMed and even the FDA show that this food does cause these disorders. Every time I look at the data, I'm forced to ask myself, why hasn't' the FDA, WHA, or the ADA condemned this food? These agencies have to know what's going on, yet they refuse to act. Who is blocking this action? Why does *MYPlate.gov* still recommend them?

After researching my book *IT'S TIME FOR A CURE*, I've learned that this food is at the base of all of the diseases listed above, forcing me to ask, why hasn't the FDA or the WHF warned us of this food? The only reason I can come up with is that it is being protected from prosecution by the industry that provides the crop seed for the farmer as well as the drugs to combat arthritis caused by what their seed grows into.

After finding this, I don't wonder at all why the FDA isn't protecting us. It's because they're protecting Monsanto as Michael Taylor was their deputy commissioner since 2010; *Michael R. Taylor is an American lawyer. Since*

2010 he has been the Deputy Commissioner for Foods at the United States Food and Drug Administration

His past associations include 4 years with Monsanto. Do you wonder if he left with any stock options? Does he still have an interest in Monsanto's business? Their offices are loaded with people as such, corrupting the integrity of our food chain.

From Wikipedia;

Between 1996 and 2000, after briefly returning to King & Spalding, Taylor worked for Monsanto as a Vice President for Public Policy. In 1999, a lawsuit (Alliance For Bio-Integrity v. Shalala) and GAO report revealed considerable disagreement within the FDA concerning decisions about biotechnology products made during Taylor's tenure. The lawsuit and report also said that Taylor had recused himself from matters related to Monsanto's BGH and had "never sought to influence the thrust or content" of the agency's policies on Monsanto's products.

Was this following study something that he didn't want to be exposed? Or was he worried about any of the other 11,750 studies done on glycation, the end result of glucose consumption, or carb consumption?

From PubMed's study; *Characterization of Proteins from Grain of Different Bread and Durum Wheat Genotypes: "Wheat is unique among the edible grains because wheat flour has the protein complex called "gluten" that can be formed into the dough with the rheological properties required for the production of leavened bread. The rheological properties of gluten are needed not only for bread production, but also in the wider range of foods that can only be made from wheat, viz., noodles, pasta, pocket bread, pastries, cookies, and other products. The gluten proteins consist of monomeric gliadins and polymeric glutenins. Glutenins and gliadins are recognized as the major wheat storage proteins, constituting about 75–85% of the total grain proteins with a ratio of about 1:1 in common or bread wheat and they tend to be rich in asparagine, glutamine, arginine or proline but very low in nutritionally important amino acids lysine, tryptophan, and methionine."*

"Very low in nutritionally important amino acids" interests me. Amino acids are proteins. When you take away the protein, you're left with little else but carbohydrates. This fact combined with the fact that gliadins have been shown to provoke the body to release anti-gliadin antibodies, which also have been shown to have the ability to attach themselves to Purkinje cells in the cerebellum, make this food suspect, at the least.

When an anti-gliadin antibody attaches itself to a cell in the cerebellum, the brain renders that cell useless and discards it. Although many parts of your brain can grow new cells to replace discarded cells, this area of the brain can't. That means whenever an anti-gliadin antibody attaches itself to a Purkinje cell, that part of the brain never comes back. Yes, that does mean brain damage for those who release these anti-gliadin antibodies.

The question this brings up is how many of us release these antibodies? Judging from the amount of Alzheimer's disease invading the civilized world, I would say a majority of people display this form of intolerance....a rather large majority. The next question this generates is, am I one of them? Are you one of them? I found out that I am. Have you yet?

42,657 deaths each day worldwide from cardiovascular disease

Heart disease kills more people every year than any other single cause. Over 42,000 people die from this disease every day and the only reason it exists is the high amount of sugar we put into our bodies. It brings about the glycation that **ECC** is responsible for and it's this glycation that is responsible 42,000 deaths from cardiovascular disease every day. That's 1,680 Americans every day. That's 33 people for every state every day, dying from a cardiovascular disease caused by nothing other than ECC, Excessive Carbohydrate Consumption.

But that's not all it is responsible for. We have to look at Alzheimer's disease and dementia. We have to consider cancer, and we have to worry about the amount of high blood pressure and high cholesterol ECC is responsible for. All of these disorders are money producing the diseases that this industry generates, simply for the sake of profit. It's this profit that is killing everyone

13,698 daily deaths globally from Alzheimer disease

13.698 die each day, worldwide, due to Alzheimer disease. That amounts to over 500 deaths daily in the US, which means that at least 20 people in this country will die this hour alone, due to Alzheimer disease. Nothing contributes to Alzheimer disease as much as bread consumption. It's the starchy carbs that break down to glucose, and it's the glucose that glycates the cholesterol and protein that builds up the plaque and inflammation in your blood that leads to Alzheimer disease, cancer, arthritis, Atherosclerosis as well as most all other CVDs, as well as hypertension and high cholesterol.

11,232 deaths daily from cancer worldwide

11,232 people die every day globally due to some form of cancer and with all the evidence available that wheat contributes to the spread of multiple forms of cancer, why hasn't the FDA made any statements about the dangers this food presents to the human body. Evidence shows this devastating effects going back to the bones of earliest cavemen that have been discovered.

I recently watched a Nova program on a 5,000-year-old iceman mummy that had been frozen in an ice flow until he was discovered in 1991. They found remnants of einkorn wheat in his upper digestive tract suggesting his last meal was bread made from the flour of einkorn wheat. His bones also showed "disease of a modern lifestyle", as they like to call it. What is this disease of a modern lifestyle? Arthritis! This is evidence of the glycation that occurred in this man from eating the carb-loaded grain from einkorn wheat. Even as difficult as it was to digest einkorn wheat at that time, due to its fibrous nature, it still did the same damage then, that it does today to everyone who continues to eat this food.

Copied from NOVA on PBS concerning a 5,000-year-old frozen mummy;

"OEGGL RECONSTRUCTED THE ICEMAN'S LAST MEAL FROM HIS MICROSCOPIC ANALYSIS OF A TINY SAMPLE REMOVED FROM THE MUMMY'S TRANSVERSE COLON, THE PART OF THE INTESTINE JUST BEYOND THE STOMACH. WHEN THE ICEMAN WAS DISCOVERED IN 1991, X-RAYS AND CAT-SCANS OF THE CORPSE REVEALED THAT HIS INTERNAL ORGANS HAD SHRUNKEN SO DRASTICALLY IN THE 5,300 YEARS IN THE GLACIER THAT DR. DIETER ZUR NEDDEN, THE RADIOLOGIST WHO EXAMINED THE IMAGES, COULD BARELY DISTINGUISH THEM. INSTEAD OF FILLING THE CHEST CAVITY WITH THEIR BILLOWY WHITE FORM, THE LUNGS LOOKED LIKE WISPS OF CLOUDS.

BUT AT THE TOP OF THE COLON, ZUR NEDDEN MADE OUT A SLIGHT BULGE, WHICH THE RADIOLOGIST SUSPECTED WAS A CLUMP OF HALF-PROCESSED FOOD. THE PROGRESS OF THE FOOD INDICATED THAT THE ICEMAN HAD LAST EATEN ABOUT EIGHT HOURS BEFORE HE DIED, POSSIBLY OF HYPOTHERMIA, ON THE HAUSLABJOCH PASS, WHICH CUTS OVER THE MAIN ALPINE RIDGE DIVIDING AUSTRIA FROM ITALY AT 10,500 FEET ABOVE SEA LEVEL.

NOT UNTIL SEVERAL YEARS AFTER THE DISCOVERY DID THE INNSBRUCK SCIENTISTS FINALLY CUT A HOLE INTO THE MUMMY, INSERT AN ENDOSCOPE, AND SNIP OUT ABOUT .004 OUNCES FROM THE COLON. DR. WERNER PLATZER, THE UNIVERSITY OF INNSBRUCK ANATOMIST THEN IN CHARGE OF RESEARCH ON THE CORPSE, GAVE .0016 OUNCES MILLIGRAMS OF THE MATERIAL TO OEGGL, WHO HAD ALREADY BEEN STUDYING THE RICH BOTANICAL FINDS FROM THE SITE.

POLLEN PROVIDED A SNAPSHOT OF THE ENVIRONMENT THE ICEMAN WAS EXPOSED TO IN THE HOURS BEFORE HIS DEATH

OEGGL'S SAMPLE WAS BARELY THE SIZE OF HIS LITTLE FINGERNAIL. UNDER THE MICROSCOPE, HE QUICKLY IDENTIFIED THE FLAKE-LIKE, SEMI-DIGESTED

MATERIAL THAT MADE UP THE BULK OF THE SAMPLE AS **EINKORN**, THE MOST IMPORTANT **WHEAT** OF THE NEOLITHIC, THE PERIOD OF PREHISTORY IN WHICH PEOPLE LIVED IN SEMI-PERMANENT SETTLEMENTS AND SURVIVED BY AGRICULTURE AND KEEPING ANIMALS. THE DISCOVERY OF EINKORN, WHICH DOES NOT OCCUR NATURALLY IN EUROPE, IN THE ICEMAN'S INTESTINAL TRACT, SUGGESTED THAT HE HAD CONTACT WITH AN AGRICULTURAL COMMUNITY. THE DOMINANCE OF BRAN IN THE SAMPLE LED OEGGL TO BELIEVE THAT THE WHEAT HAD BEEN FINELY GROUND INTO MEAL AND MADE INTO BREAD, RATHER THAN EATEN AS A PORRIDGE, WHERE THE GRAINS WOULD HAVE BEEN EATEN WHOLE AND FOUND IN LARGER PIECES IN THE COLON. BUT THE BREAD WOULD HAVE BEEN LITTLE LIKE MODERN BREAD. IN ORDER TO GET BREAD TO RISE WHEN YEAST IS ADDED, THE WHEAT GRAINS MUST CONTAIN A HIGH LEVEL OF GLUTEN, WHICH LENDS THE DOUGH A DURABLE ELASTICITY AND THEREFORE HOLDS THE POCKETS OF AIR. EINKORN HAS LOW LEVELS OF GLUTEN, SO THE BREAD MADE WITH IT, WAS PROBABLY HARD, SOMEWHAT LIKE A CRACKER, AND RATHER TOUGH ON THE TEETH.

USING AN ELECTRON MICROSCOPE OEGGL ALSO SPOTTED TINY PARTICLES OF CHARCOAL ATTACHED TO THE BRAN, PROBABLY REMNANTS OF THE BAKING PROCESS ON A HOT ROCK, OR NEXT TO A FIRE. IN ADDITION TO THE EINKORN, THE CELLS OF AT LEAST ONE OTHER PLANT, POSSIBLY SOME HERB, WERE PRESENT IN THE SAMPLE, AND OEGGL CONCLUDED THAT THEY, TOO, HAD BEEN PART OF HIS MEAL. HE ALSO FOUND A TINY MUSCLE FIBER AND A BURNED BIT OF BONE, EVIDENCE THAT THE ICEMAN MIGHT ALSO HAVE EATEN A MEAT. WHAT KIND OF MEAT OEGGL CANNOT YET SAY, NOR CAN HE DETERMINE HOW MUCH OF THE MEAL THE SAMPLE REPRESENTED. NOT EVERYTHING PASSING THROUGH THE ICEMAN'S GUT HAD BEEN SWALLOWED INTENTIONALLY, OR WAS EVEN DESIRABLE. OEGGL ALSO FOUND THE EGGS OF THE HUMAN WHIPWORM. MANY PEOPLE ALIVE TODAY WHO DO NOT LIVE IN AREAS WITH FLUSH TOILETS ALSO CARRY THE WORM, WHICH CAN CAUSE UNPLEASANT SYMPTOMS LIKE STOMACH ACHE AND DIARRHEA, OR EVEN LEAD TO MALNUTRITION. THE SCIENTISTS HAVE NO WAY OF KNOWING WHETHER THE ICEMAN HAD ANY SUCH COMPLAINTS.

SCIENTISTS MAY NEVER KNOW WHAT PROMPTED THE ICEMAN TO LEAVE THE RELATIVELY HOSPITABLE VALLEY WITH NO WATER OR FOOD TO SPEAK OF. THE SAMPLE ALSO CONTAINED MANY DIFFERENT VARIETIES OF POLLEN, WHOSE STRANGE AND BEAUTIFUL FORMS OEGGL SAW UNDER THE ELECTRON MICROSCOPE. THOUGH SOME PEOPLES ARE KNOWN TO EAT POLLEN, OEGGL BELIEVED THAT THE QUANTITY IN HIS COLON WAS TOO SMALL TO REPRESENT A MEAL. INSTEAD, THE POLLEN ACCIDENTALLY ENDED UP IN THE MAN'S STOMACH BECAUSE THEY EITHER HAD LANDED IN FOOD OR WATER HE INGESTED, OR WERE INHALED AND BECAME TRAPPED IN HIS SALIVA WHICH HE THEN SWALLOWED. SCIENTISTS HAD LONG WONDERED WHERE THE ICEMAN WAS COMING FROM AND WHERE HE WAS HEADED, BUT UNTIL THE DISCOVERY OF THE POLLEN INSIDE THE CORPSE, NO SCIENTIST HAD ANY CONVINCING DOCUMENTATION FOR HIS LAST DAY. BUT THE POLLEN PROVIDED A SNAPSHOT OF THE ENVIRONMENT THE ICEMAN WAS EXPOSED TO IN THE HOURS BEFORE HIS DEATH.

This feature originally appeared on the site for the Nova program *ICE*

MUMMIES.

Although not shown in this excerpt, the Iceman did show signs of modern day disease in his bones. it was evident mostly around his joints in the form of arthritis. This arthritis is directly due to his diet of einkorn wheat.

As it does now, it did it then. The glucose glycates the cholesterol it comes in contact with, causing arthritis. It did so then, as it does now. It just did it slower, due to the indigestibility of the einkorn wheat. But it happened, never-the-less.

The damage it did at that time was much less than what it does now. This is due to the lack of fiber it comes with, in today's strains of wheat, mostly the common bread wheat made of Triticum aestivum, and, spelled, rye and emmer. It also comes from more glutinous wheat like durum as well.

Even though arthritis seldom kills its victim, the damage it does doesn't go away, ever. It's stuck to you like paint on a wall and you can't scrape it off. Most of the today's wheat has more gluten protein than it's ever had in its history, making it gluier and stickier, which makes it that much more dangerous, as this is what builds up the plaque in your system and you already know what damage plaque does. This points to the fact this food which is eaten on a daily basis does so little damage incrementally to the consumer that it's never noticed until it's too late. The disease has already manifested itself and the price is now being paid for a lifetime of consumption.

Perhaps the biggest question this brings up is, with all of this information available for this many years, why hasn't the FDA warned us that this food has these capabilities to do this kind of damage to the human body. Should the public be able to make an informed decision as to whether or not to continue to eat this food? Or should the FDA continue to ignore the evidence and fail to even let the public know what this food does? The question I want to ask, was and is there outside influence in their decision to not expose this information?

The evidence is piling up. The FDA, nor the USDA can't hide their complicity much longer.

Someone is trying to hide this information. They want to leave it up to an uneducated public to automatically know what these studies have shown. In whose best interest would it be to keep this information hidden? Whose business would hurt the most if bread and corn and wheat products all of a sudden became taboo? The grain industry? Monsanto? The more I look into this, the more it spells out cover-up and because this is how the FDA treats this, it creates a lot of fear in me as to how healthy the rest of our food supply is.

I contend that The FDA has to know of the damage these grains do to the body when ingested, so why do they allow these industries to continue to peddle their wares as if they're healthy? (This is the definition of inside influence.)

Food, Inc. is a 2008 American documentary film directed by filmmaker Robert Kenner. The academy award-nominated film examines corporate farming in the United States, concluding that agribusiness produces food that is unhealthy, in a way that is environmentally harmful and abusive to both animals and employees. The film is narrated by Michael Pollan and Eric Schlosser

The film received positive responses and was nominated for several awards, including the academy award and the independent spirit awards in 2009, both for best documentary feature.

The film's first segment examines the industrial production of meat (chicken, beef, and pork), calling it inhumane and economically and environmentally unsustainable. The second segment looks at the industrial production of grains and vegetables (primarily corn and soybeans), again labeling this economically and environmentally unsustainable. The film's third and final segment is about the economic and legal power, such as food labeling regulations, of the major food companies, the profits of which are based on supplying cheap but contaminated food, the heavy use of petroleum-based chemicals (largely pesticides and fertilizers), and the promotion of unhealthy food consumption habits by the American public. It shows companies like Walmart transitioning towards organic foods as that industry is booming in the recent health movement.

Monsanto, the USDA and the FDA

FOOD, INC is an eye-opening documentary that deals with the agricultural industry's influence in the USDA and the FDA, concentrating on the meatpacking industry's influence. In 2008 the Chief of Staff for the USDA was a former chief lobbyist for the beef industry. The head of the FDA was a former executive vice president for the national food processors Association. A majority of the staff at both the FDA and the USDA came from Monsanto or its subsidiaries, posing clear conflicts of interests when it comes to protecting consumers. These industries; Monsanto, Bayer, Syngenta have spread their influence throughout the offices and agencies of the USDA and the FDA and are ultimately responsible for more death and disease than all violence, which includes war and crime, as well as all automobile accidents, all other addictions, including heroin, amphetamines, and alcohol. This addiction can be blamed for every other addiction that exists, simply because of the control, this addiction has over your hormones combined with the fact that this addiction was forced upon you right after birth.

Food, Inc talks about the revolving door between Monsanto's corporate offices and the various regulatory agencies that are supposed to protect us, the consumer. Donald Rumsfeld was CEO of Searle, which was owned by Monsanto. You know of his close ties to the Bush White House, John Ashcroft (Missouri Senator) received record donations from Monsanto. According to *Food, Inc.* for 25 years our government agencies that are set up to protect us were dominated by the industry they regulate. This is how Monsanto self-regulates. They pretty much own the gov't agencies. That makes it convenient to keep control of your drugs and how much you pay for them.

Justice Clarence Thomas was a Monsanto attorney prior to being named a Supreme Court Justice, which wouldn't matter too much except for the fact that he wrote the decision the court made, that allows Monsanto to prohibit farmers (both contracted and uncontracted) from cleaning their own seeds to use for next year's planting (according to *Food, Inc*).

Something as natural as a seed is what the Supreme Court has allowed Monsanto to patent. The consequence of this has been disastrous for the farmer. It's been far worse for the consumer. Now, Monsanto controls all the food you buy, if you're buying the carbs their crops are made into. Most all seed companies are owned by Monsanto. If a farmer wants to grow a crop, they have to buy seed for that crop from Monsanto. This is unless you're old enough to have your own seed that you've never bought. You've just kept re-using your crop from last year for this year's seed. This requires cleaning a portion of your crop to use as seed for next year's crop. This is how farmers improved their own crops. They would pick out the best section of their fields to clean for next year's crops.

This is where the problem begins for these farmers. Seed cleaners used to have thriving businesses in the Midwest. Now, few if any of them exist. This is an industry that's been put to death by Monsanto and their patented seeds. Monsanto guarantees their demise by threatening any farmers that use their services, legal action. This is to inhibit any farmer from cleaning their own seeds. (Monsanto uses the patent clause in their contracts to prosecute farmers for growing their GMO seeds when in all actuality their crops have been cross-pollinated by their neighbor's GMO crops.)

Say goodbye to homegrown in your food. It all belongs to Monsanto now. Don't forget though, they also made your Celebrex.

Crops that are grown in an open field are open to the environment. Being open to the environment leaves them open to cross-pollination. This cross-pollination happens when neighboring field's GMO crops and portions of a non-GMO field get contaminated with GMO cross-pollination. Monsanto makes their farmers sign a "no clean" contract, saying that they can't clean a portion of their seed to save for planting next year. If caught doing so, they're open for prosecution. However, the farmer growing his own seed that's been contaminated by GMO cross-pollination is now open to prosecution by Monsanto, your food provider.

This puts your food if you're eating carbs, completely under the control of the same company that controls the drug industry that treats you for the conditions their foods give you. This is the glucose ruse, the ultimate carb haul, the emanate destroyer of health and life. This may be the superlative of corporate chicanery, your health risked, all for the sake of profit, and what drives profit? The ~~desire~~ hunger for security drives the desire for profit. It's the same hunger as that for food. It a hunger for security, it's an impulse to stay alive and hopefully make life easier to ensure a longer life.

It would be OK if you had a choice in the matter. But you didn't. (Would you choose an addiction, if you had a choice?) This one has been forced upon you just like it was me and if I could break the cycle, with all the issues I have, you can too.

These industries and agencies are directly responsible for over 950,000 deaths each and every year. That total continues to climb and it will continue until everyone decides, like me, that it's time for a cure.

Decisions have been made in the past that clearly benefited industry while presenting clear dangers to humans. By allowing contaminated food with worthless nutritional values or food contaminated by bacteria to sneak into our food supply, as well as by polluting our rivers and lakes in the process, with contaminated groundwater from runoff from chemical fertilizers, pesticides and herbicides, Monsanto has probably contributed more to the damage of mankind than any other one entity. This is the primary reason this is unsustainable and has to be changed.

It all starts with the grain industry, along with our insatiable appetites for high starch and sugary foods (which is all forced upon us by this industry) the corn producers, the wheat growers, and the crop seed companies owned by Monsanto, Novartis, Syngenta, Bayer ET AL. Because their food requires treatment with medications that this industry controls, they have full control over what happens inside your body when you bend to their will and buy their products.

The Iowa Corn Fed Beef Controversy

The grain industry in Iowa promoted *"Iowa Corn Fed Beef"*, to sell more corn, their largest industry. This had multiple, unforeseen consequences that not only damaged our food supply, but it polluted our resources more than what could have ever been foreseen.

The increase in industrial beef production that this promotion has generated has damaged the quality of the beef as well as damage the environment with the pesticides and herbicides needed for growing the corn to use as feed for the cattle. This has acted as a double whammy for our environment.

The huge cattle farms act as methane farms contributing more to global warming than much of anything else in the environment. On top of that, the chemicals sprayed on the fields of corn that's to be used for feed ultimately put these chemicals into our food supply as well as washing off the crops to contaminate groundwater and runoff into the streams and rivers polluting drinking water. This led to multiple outbreaks of cancer in downstream communities.

The cattle eat these glyphosate herbicide infected grains, (mostly soy and corn) which infects the meat which you eat. This is basically putting this enzyme changing chemicals in your body. Can you see how the ingestion of enzyme changing chemicals could have an impact on your health? This is just a taste (no pun intended) of what this industry is putting our society through. How safe would you consider your food is from these chemicals?

A lot of this feed corn that's been genetically modified to accept the Roundup weedkiller that's been sprayed on it, finds its way through the food supply into your processed foods, to make ingredients for foods that you commonly eat. I'll bet you didn't know you were buying cancer when you bought those corn chips last time, did you? How about that power bar or soy milk? If you're not reading labels on the food you're buying, how do you know you're not subjecting your body to this damage?

Or how about when you bought that formula or medicine for your baby? The #1 or #2 ingredient in many Similac infant formulas and Pedialyte is corn syrup and corn syrup solids right behind water. Often the second or third ingredient is soy protein. Arguably the 2 heaviest sprayed crops in our food supply are soybeans and corn, ensuring your baby's diet is herbicide laden. Do you think that could cause some future need for further medication for your baby, in the future? And don't forget, drug use always leads to more and more drug use, especially when the drug is basically sugar. The only thing that can stop it is to either, quit the carbs and go keto, or die prematurely of any disease of your body's choice.

Because of our propensity to feed our addiction to sugar (which includes all grains), the products that this industry has devised to get us to eat more of their junk food, are putting everyone who is suckered into this cycle, in the hospital with serious disorders. You should know the range of disorders this incurs by now, from arthritis to cancer to hypertension to CVDs, anything involving inflammation including all dementia. The scale is staggering. The toll is staggering.

This is clearly a case where self-policing doesn't work. It's taking its toll on Americans, currently at a rate of 196 of us every hour, because it isn't working. From all ECC caused forms of death, this glucose addiction is costing our country 959,993 premature deaths, every year that could have been prevented by a simple change of diet. That's 2,630 mothers and fathers every day or 109 family members every hour. Evidence can be seen in the number of heart disease deaths, cancer deaths, Alzheimer's deaths, and this doesn't mention all the pain, discomfort, and drug abuse that comes along with the disease. All of this is due to the pain and discomfort the disease inflicts.

When I consider how close I was to suicide because of my pain and seeing no way out of it, I have to consider many suicides as being caused by carbohydrates now. If carbs weren't at the root of my pain, I definitely wouldn't have been as close to suicide as I was, for I would not have had as much pain. That and the fact that sugar does mess with your emotions by messing with your hormones makes it much easier to see how suicide could be considered caused by ECC. Depression is another manifestation of glucose addiction, I know, I was there. It's become clear to me that if you don't die of old age, and I mean really old age, (as in 100 years old or older) your death is going to be a result of your addiction.

Although this is nice for the profits of Monsanto, Syngenta and Bayer who also make drugs that treat the diseases their foods cause; it's leading our country down a path of destruction that we'll never recover from if you keep eating the food they keep pushing you to eat. They are counting on the addiction that they've inflicted upon the American people as well as the world to pad their profits and boost the influence, both commercially and politically.

This industry's desire to make certain that sugar gets into as much baby food as they can pack it into, to make sure that every baby who eats it becomes addicted to it, making them lifetime **users** of their poison. This unwilling addiction to sugar, by the public at large, has brought this industry to a level of evil that's never been seen in any industry. This industry is so intent on keeping us addicted to its lure, simply to increase their profits, that they are now responsible for over 65,753 deaths, worldwide daily. Yes, I said 65,753 deaths daily. If this doesn't bother you, then you have no conscience. Yes, this is something to be appalled about and appalled I am and you should be too. This is simply more proof that it's time for a cure.

It was recently revealed that the sugar industry took steps to cover up the reports of damage that their food offered, so why wouldn't it make sense that this closely related industry, the grain industry, would take those same steps to cover up the same information about what their foods provided? Was this another case of the industry policing itself and its watchdog, as well? Does this make a valid argument for the self-policing of corporate entities like this, instead of government regulations? This is the epitome of corporate propaganda generated to bolster profits by building their influence in the regulatory departments that are responsible for our health. This is my worst dream come true, someone else controlling my health by controlling my food.

For the sake of profit, this industry has poisoned not only us the consumer, but the space we have to live in as well, as they've contaminated our environment and condemned our society to a cycle of dependence that can only end with a premature death. There is an alternative. You can always join me and go keto. It'll not only save your life, it will extend it.

Our health is at stake here and we've allowed the USDA and the FDA to escape judgment. That in my estimation is borderline criminal. 2,893 deaths nationally, each day from CVDs, cancer, and Alzheimer disease combined. All three of these disorders are directly due to ECC, excessive carbohydrate consumption, which can be controlled. That's enough people to wipe out 4 towns, the same size I grew up in. That's unconscionable and we let it happen. Shame on us, for allowing this ruse to continue.

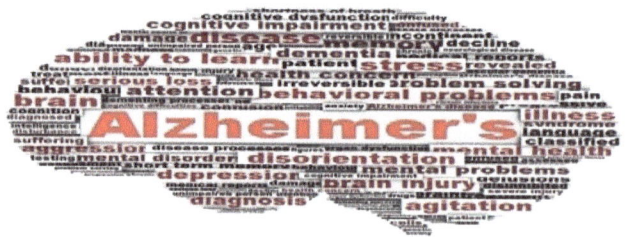

We have direct control of these disorders. We don't have to let this continue, but we do, simply to feed our addiction. We have a societal addiction to glucose. Because it's not just sugar, it's what breaks down into glucose, and that includes not only sugar but all carbohydrates that break down to their most basic molecule, glucose. It's our addiction to this glucose that clouds our judgment, masks our emotions, and controls our desires by gumming up the neurons in our brains every time we eat this food. This is exactly what makes it addictive and hands total control over to the glucose, every time you eat it.

Yes, we do have full control over this, and you can stop it. We have to stop the celebration of our individual addiction, to stop the addiction on a societal level. We need to un-brainwash ourselves and learn to see pain every time we see bread, pasta, cereal, and sugar because that's all it brings.

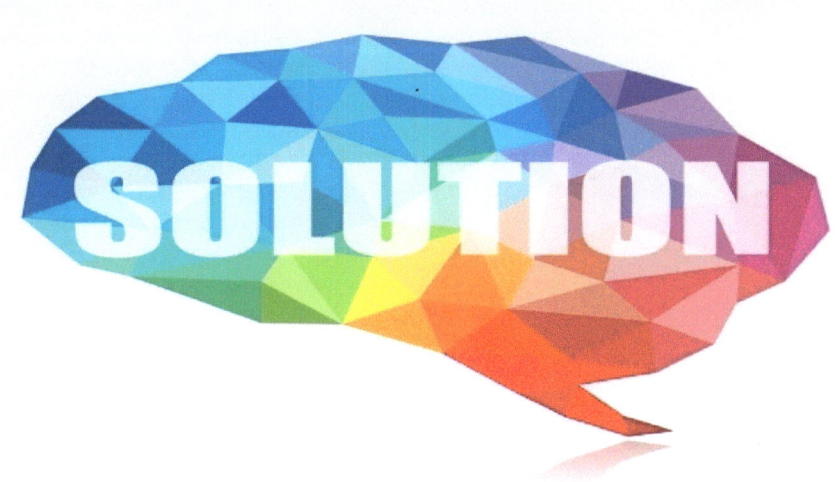

You have the power to stop it and by stopping it, it gives you far more power, than what you ever could have imagined you would have.

CHAPTER 9
USDA'S INVOLVEMENT

With the same commingling of execs and offices of the USDA and Monsanto, as between the FDA and Monsanto, Monsanto has set itself up to be producer and regulator in full control over all of the food that we are forced to put on our tables. That is if you're forced to eat at a restaurant or buy food at a grocery store. If you're one of those people, your food is more than likely, a product of Monsanto. It's also a product of Monsanto's chemicals, chiefly their herbicide Roundup, a glyphosate herbicide that inhibits how enzymes work in the environment as well as your body.

That wouldn't be so bad if Monsanto didn't force all farmers to grow their crop seed each and every year. That gives them full control over every muffin you sink your teeth into, even those bran muffins, the ones that are supposed to be so healthy.

What Monsanto knows that they're not telling the USDA, is that the corn, wheat, and soybeans that their farmers grow for us are at the root of most all glycation that occurs in the body. What they're afraid of the USDA knowing, is that this glycation is at the root of all modern diseases, from atherosclerosis to hypertension, from arthritis to IBS or irritable bowel syndrome, to dementia including Alzheimer's disease and Parkinson's disease. All of these diseases and disorders are treated by the drug industry that Monsanto owned as well. That's what's scary...very scary. The company that's responsible for your food is the same company that treats you for the ailments their food brings. To me that's criminal. Now, Bayer wants to buy out Monsanto. What do you think that will do to your food supply? Bayer is a German company, you know.

Monsanto doesn't want either the USDA or the FDA to be too aware of what their food does, yet all of the studies mentioned above are available through PubMed. If I have access to these studies, I know they do as well. What don't I know is what do they refuse to look at them? They only have to look at a few. I found two or three damning studies on the first page of search returns for the term, glycation. Glycation has a nasty tendency to muck up everything in the body that blood effects. Monsanto doesn't want the USDA or the FDA to realize this. Their practice of striving for total control over our food source drives the profits of their crop seed companies, (of which they're dozens). Having that control over our food gives them control over our drug use, as it's their food that makes us sick. That makes us require their medications to treat the disease their food gives those who eat it.

They've tried denying that their food is as dangerous as it is by publishing their own research reports showing different results that "prove" their food is healthy when it's not. It's obvious that they don't want this information known by either the USDA or the FDA. Fortunately for Monsanto, they already have they own retired execs running the FDA and the USDA. Apparently, it's not in their best interest to make this information known to the public. I'm sure they fear the consequences of their actions, for producing a food this dangerous. I would be if I were them.

With all the agencies the USDA has control over, it's no wonder that they can't see that the food they recommend we eat, has had more studies done on the glycation of it than any other food. We've learned that glycation is the real poisoning of America, and with glycation being involved in every modern disease known to man (simply because of the glycation is caused), glycation is something that our food industry should be working to stem as it's this glycation that's at the root of all "modern" diseases.

FYI fact: There were 50,000 food safety inspections in 1972. That was reduced to just over 9,000 in 2008.

If there were only 9000 in 2008, reduced from 50,000 in 1972, when the threat level was much lower, the FDA is only succeeding at failing us on an unprecedented basis. I'm sure this is due to funding cutbacks from the government but I'm also sure it involves something related to departmental offices being run by corporate management brought in from corporations they're supposed to regulate, proving once again that money talks and (unfortunately) the bottom line is what wins here and the bottom line is greed. If the USDA and the FDA can allow a food this dangerous through its monitoring, I'm afraid to even think about what else has snuck through? The beef industry has already displayed their contempt for regulation through the mass production of beef that their industry is responsible for, especially in the last 30 years. (Including that beef that's imported from Paraguay, the most GMO soy loaded feed made for feedlots.) That's a whole other story about how this industry is ruining the lives of our South American neighbor by poisoning their crops and the lives of their farmers. This is just so you can have cheap beef.

According to their Website, USDA.gov their agencies and offices include the following (I'm listing all of them so you'll know the enormity of this agency). It has to be enormous, 19 agencies and 17 offices, all designed to protect you. Your health is at stake and a majority of this Departments' agencies and offices are failing to keep your food safe for consumption.

AGENCIES:

Agricultural Marketing Service (AMS)

AMS facilitates the strategic marketing of agricultural products in domestic and international markets while ensuring fair trading practices and promoting a competitive and efficient marketplace. AMS constantly works to develop new marketing services to increase customer satisfaction. It's responsible for developing quality grade standards for agricultural commodities, administering marketing regulatory programs, marketing agreements and orders, and making food purchases for USDA food assistance programs.
Program and Service Highlights:
Agricultural Transportation
Country of Origin Labeling
Farmers Market
Farmers Market Promotion Program
Federal-State Marketing Improvement Program
Food Purchases
Grade Standards
Local Food Marketing
Market News Reports
National Organic Program

I have to wonder if they check the quality and safety of the grain they're approving for consumption, whether it's for livestock feed or human consumption. Are they aware that what they're approving is contaminated? I'm curious as to how they grade this substandard grain that's putting so many people in the hospital? Evidently they not detecting the Roundup that's it's laden with.

Agricultural Research Service (ARS)

ARS is USDA's principal in-house research agency. ARS leads America towards a better future through agricultural research and information. (ARS) works to ensure that Americans have reliable, adequate supplies of high-quality food and other agricultural products. ARS accomplishes its goals through scientific discoveries that help solve problems in crop and livestock production and protection, human nutrition, and the interaction of agriculture and the environment.
Programs and service highlights:
National Research
International Research
Research Partnerships and Technology
Research Locations
National Agricultural Library

The question I'd like to ask this department is how much research do you pay attention to when you recommend what food to eat. Does your research cover the effects of grains after they've been consumed? They claim to be interested in nutrition. Are they? Or are they interested in their own bottom line with their stock options with Monsanto?

Animal and Plant Health Inspection Service (APHIS)

APHIS provides leadership in ensuring the health and care of animals and plants. The agency improves agricultural productivity and competitiveness and contributes to the national economy and the public health.
(APHIS) is responsible for protecting and promoting U.S. agricultural health, administering the Animal Welfare Act, and carrying out wildlife damage management activities.
Programs and service highlights:
Cattle Disease Information
Plant Health Import Permits
Plant Export Certificates and Forms
Animal Health Permits
Animal and Animal Product Export Information
Wood Packaging Material
- Animal Welfare Act (AWA) Licensing and Registration

Center for Nutrition Policy and Promotion (CNPP)

CNPP works to improve the health and well-being of Americans by developing and promoting dietary guidance that links scientific research to the nutrition needs of consumers.
(CNPP) works to improve the health and well-being of Americans by developing and promoting dietary guidance that links scientific research to the nutrition needs of consumers.
Programs and service highlights:
ChooseMyPlate
MyPlate Blast Off Game and Information for Children
SuperTracker and Other Tools
Dietary Guidelines for Americans
Healthy Eating Index
Nutrition Insights
These are the offices that are supposed to ensure that the food you eat on a daily basis, no matter where it comes from or where you buy it (grocery store or restaurant), is going to keep you healthy. Have you ever considered the value of their work or the quality of the food they approve for your table? With the high rates of Atherosclerosis, cancer, inflammatory diseases and dementia, it appears that they are failing on a massive scale.

(Unless you were looking at it from a corporate point of view where this is an investors dream, this is a consumer's nightmare.) Regardless of how unscrupulous this is, it's going to continue to happen as long as this agency recommends the consumption of these foods.

Myplate.gov, which is administered by the CNPP, has replaced the food pyramid for our dietary guidelines. Myplate.gov is now our dietary guidelines and it still insists that grains remain a part of our diet. I've asked them about this and have received one reply from someone who didn't even know what glycation is or what it is responsible for. I'm still waiting for my reply for that and another email I've not so recently sent them.

Economic Research Service (ERS)
ERS is USDA's principal social science research agency. Each year, ERS communicates research results and socioeconomic indicators via briefings, analyses for policymakers and their staffs, market analysis updates, and major reports. (ERS) provides economic research and information to inform public and private decision making on economic and policy issues related to agriculture, food, natural resources, and rural America. Through a broad range of products, ERS research provides not only facts, but also expert economic analysis of many critical issues facing farmers, agribusiness, consumers, and policymakers. ERS expertise helps these stakeholders conduct business, formulate policy, or just learn about agriculture, food, natural resources, and rural America.
Programs and service highlights:
Food and Nutrition Assistance
Food Safety
Farm Sector Income & Finances
Food Markets and Prices
Natural Resources and Environment
Agricultural Markets and Trade
Rural Communities and Development
Farm and Commodity Policy
Agricultural R&D and Productivity
Amber Waves Magazine
State Fact Sheets
Commodity Outlook Reports

These are the offices regulate the safety of our food. I wonder if they are aware of the dangers of grains in the food supply. One would think that they are, but with 109 people dying every hour, I have to wonder.

Farm Service Agency (FSA)
The Farm Service Agency implements agricultural policy, administers credit and loan programs, and manages conservation, commodity, disaster and farm marketing programs through a national network of offices. (FSA)

administers farm commodity, crop insurance, credit, environmental, conservation, and emergency assistance programs for farmers and ranchers.
Programs and service highlights:
Farm Loan Programs
Disaster Assistance
Price Support
Conservation Programs
Daily Market Prices
Commodity Procurement
This is the agency that watches over the farmer and their needs and concerns. Their interest doesn't concern the safety of the food we eat or how nutritious it is. They're simply concerned about the farmer's ability to grow it. They offer the assistance programs that help fund the industry.

Food and Nutrition Service (FNS)

FNS increases food security and reduces hunger in partnership with cooperating organizations by providing children and low-income people access to food, a healthy diet, and nutrition education in a manner that supports American agriculture and inspires public confidence. (FNS) administers the food and nutrition assistance programs in the U.S. Department of Agriculture. FNS provides children and needy families with better access to food and a more healthful diet through its programs and nutrition education efforts.
Programs and service highlights:
Women, Infant, and Children (WIC) Program
Supplemental Nutrition Assistance Program
School Meals
Food Distribution Programs
Disaster Assistance
Child and Adult Care Food Program
Summer Food Service Program
Farmers Markets Nutrition Programs
Nutrition Education

This is the agency that makes sure the disadvantaged have an adequate food supply. One of their major concerns is to distribute the grains that are used in our food supply to those who don't have the ability to purchase their own. This ensures that everyone who lives in this disadvantaged lifestyle doesn't get the proper nutrition they need to sustain a healthy living and in turn, makes them dependant on the pharmaceutical industry for their future health. Don't forget that pharmaceuticals only lead to more and ultimately more pharmaceuticals. This is the never-ending cycle of dependence that this industry wants to keep the public in. This cycle is at the government expense though, and that means that we, the taxpayer get to foot the bill. It's too bad that they don't realize to conquer hunger you must first conquer the hunger cycle. If the USDA read any of the reports in the PubMed or PMC archives, they'd know that it's the grains and sugar in the diet that create hunger cycle more than anything else. If you were on a ketogenic diet, you could see the logic in this statement, to stop hunger you have to stop the hunger cycle.

This is where their logic is flawed; they think that feeding hungry people grains to fill their bellies will take care of the hunger. It won't, it will only make them hungrier; it's the law of carbohydrate consumption, it a continuous hunger cycle that you're really condemning them to. You're also condemning them to a lifetime of medication need.

Food Safety and Inspection Service (FSIS)
FSIS enhances public health and well-being by protecting the public from foodborne illness and ensuring that the nation's meat, poultry, and egg products are safe, wholesome, and correctly packaged. (FSIS) is the public health agency in the U.S. Department of Agriculture responsible for ensuring that the nation's commercial supply of meat, poultry, and egg products is safe, wholesome, and correctly labeled and packaged, as required by the Federal Meat Inspection Act, the Poultry Products Inspection Act, and the Egg Products Inspection Act.
Program and Service Highlights;
Food Safety Education
Science
Regulations and Policies
Food Recalls
Food Defense and Emergency Response
Fact Sheets
Ask Karen
If this agency had anything to do with the production of sugar and grains, I'd be in contact with them. But they don't.
It appears that this following agency ensures that the poison we grow in the US makes its way around the world to infect as many people as possible.

Foreign Agricultural Service (FAS)
FAS works to improve foreign market access for U.S. products. This USDA agency operates programs designed to build new markets and improve the competitive position of U.S. agriculture in the global marketplace. (FAS) is responsible for collecting, analyzing, and disseminating information about global supply and demand, trade trends, and market opportunities. FAS seeks improved market access for U.S. products; administers export financing and market development programs; provides export services; carries out food aid and market-related technical assistance programs; and provides linkages to world resources and international organizations.
Program and Service Highlights;

Trade News
Trade Policy
Commodity Information
Country Information
Export Programs
Food Aid Programs
Attache Reports
Export Sales Reports
North American Free Trade Agreement (NAFTA) Information
The U.S.-Central America-Dominican Republic Free Trade Agreement
(CAFTA-DR)
This may be done to ensure the viability of the pharmaceutical industry, as
all of those grains foods can only lead to more pharmaceutical needs. If you
can spread this problem around the world, what do you think that would do
for your profit margin if you're a pharmaceutical company? (Evidently,
Monsanto thinks the same way.) Maybe that's why we shouldn't allow
anyone with corporate ties in any way, to work in any of our regulatory
agencies. That would mean that government employees couldn't own any
corporate stock. I wonder how many do today. Do you think that could
constitute any conflicts of interest?

Forest Service (FS)
FS sustains the health, diversity, and productivity of the Nation's forests and
grasslands to meet the needs of present and future generations. (FS)
administers programs for applying sound conservation and utilization
practices to natural resources of the national forests and national grasslands,
for promoting these practices on all forest lands through cooperation with
states and private landowners, and for carrying out extensive forest and
range research.
Program and Service Highlights;
Fire Information
Maps and Brochures
Passes and Permits
Forest Inventory and Analysis
Forest Health Protection
Recreational Activities
Research & Development

This agency protects undeveloped land and has no control over what goes
on your table. It's the following agency that I have issues with as they inspect
the grain that's responsible for all this damage.

Grain Inspection, Packers and Stockyards Administration (GIPSA)

GIPSA facilitates the marketing of livestock, poultry, meat, cereals, oilseeds, and related agricultural products. It also promotes fair and competitive trading practices for the overall benefit of consumers and American agriculture. GIPSA ensures open and competitive markets for livestock, poultry, and meat by investigating and monitoring industry trade practices.

Programs and service highlights;

Federal Grain Inspection and Weighing Services
International Service Programs
Regulated Entities under the Packers and Stockyards Act
Packers and Stockyards Program (P&SP) Enforcement Actions
Federal Grain Inspection Service (FGIS) Providers
FGIS Handbooks and Publications
FGIS Forms
P&SP Forms
Directives and Notices
GIPSA Violation Hotline
Official U.S. Standards for Grain
Contact GIPSA

I doubt this agency even knows what they're approving when they approve this grain for consumption. If they did, they wouldn't allow this to slip right past their noses without smelling anything rotten?

National Agricultural Library (NAL)
NAL ensures and enhances access to agricultural information for a better quality of life. (NAL) provides technical information on agricultural research and related subjects to scientists, educators and farmers using computer databases; coordinates and are primary resource for a national network of state land-grant university and field libraries, and serves as the U.S. center for the international agriculture information system.
Program and Service Highlights;
Agricultural Online Access (AGRICOLA)

Agriculture Network Information Center (AgNIC)
Alternative Farming Systems Information Center (AFSIC)
Animal Welfare Information Center (AWIC)
Digital Desktop (DigiTop) for Employees
Food and Nutrition Information Center (FNIC)
Food Safety Research Information Office
Healthy Meals Resource System
National Invasive Species Information Center (NISIC)
Nutrition.gov
Rural Information Center

SNAP-Ed Connection (formerly Food Stamp Nutrition Connection)
Water Quality Information Center
WIC Works Resource System

One would think with all the departments in this agency, at least one would understand the dangers of grains. It may not be a problem of whether or not anyone knows about it, it may be a problem of anybody caring enough to do anything about it.

National Agricultural Statistics Service (NASS)
NASS serves the basic agricultural and rural data needs of the country by providing objective, important and accurate statistical information and services to farmers, ranchers, agribusinesses and public officials. This data is vital to monitoring the ever-changing agricultural sector and carrying out farm policy. (NASS) is responsible for conducting monthly and annual surveys and preparing official USDA data and estimates of production, supply, prices, and other information necessary to maintain orderly agricultural operations. NASS also conducts the census of agriculture which is currently conducted every 5 years.
Program and Service Highlights

Today's Reports
Quick Stats - Query Database by Commodity, State, and Year
Census of Agriculture
Crop Weather by State
Agricultural Charts and Maps
Agricultural Statistics by Year
Statistics by Subject
Calendar of NASS Reports

I wonder if any of their statistics show the impact that this food has had on our society as a whole, in the way it's influenced the health and medical industries with the boom of business it's created for the pharmaceutical industry. Does the government understand that the more they support the industrial GMO farming, in this case, the more it's costing them having to treat people for the disorders that this industry is imposing upon those who buy into it? How many people do you know that didn't have their toast or bagel this morning? How many of those do you think will go without a sandwich at lunch?

This is not a small problem. It exists everywhere. This is the result of politically engineering your food supply by the industry that supplies it. This is the result of self-policing. Our problem is, it's created a land of sugar junkies clamoring for their next hit, wherever they can find it. (It'll probably be the next drive through.) You unwittingly buy right into this with every Big Mac you buy. That comfort you're buying now leads only to huge amounts of discomfort in the very near future. I'll start with headaches and stomach aches. It'll end with your body's choice of disease starting with atherosclerosis and Alzheimer's, and end with cancer or cardiovascular disease. This is a cycle that must change.

I add my name to the list of many trying to get the FDA and the USDA to act on this concern. Spearheading this list were Dr. William Davis and Dr. David Perlmutter in 2010 and 2012, with their books *Wheat Belly* and *Grain Brain*. They are still trying to right this wrong. After being on both sides of this argument and experiencing all the pain that the other side has to offer, I know for a fact that the only avenue out of this dilemma, is to go to a paleo or ketogenic diet. I just wish the FDA and the USDA could understand this.

National Institute of Food and Agriculture (NIFA)
NIFA's unique mission is to advance knowledge for agriculture, the environment, human health and well-being, and communities by supporting research, education, and extension programs in the Land-Grant University System and other partner organizations. NIFA doesn't perform actual research, education, and extension but rather helps fund it at the state and local level and provides program leadership in these areas. (NIFA) is an agency within the U.S. Department of Agriculture (USDA), part of the executive branch of the Federal Government. Congress created NIFA through the Food, Conservation, and Energy Act of 2008. NIFA replaced the former Cooperative State Research, Education, and Extension Service (CSREES), which had been in existence since 1994.

I clicked on the *research* **Link to find that they're pretty proud of their involvement in peanut research, claiming that;** *North Carolina A&T research makes peanuts safer to eat.*

Maybe if they were to stop and realize that peanuts, like all legumes, are grains, they would understand that like grains, peanuts ultimately break down to glucose. They're just not cereal grains, so they inflict the harm slower, but they still have the capacity to inflict harm. Because they're harder to digest and do have more fiber than the starchy cereal grains, they impact the glycemic load much less, which is what keeps the blood glucose more even over time. Any doctor will tell you that will make you healthier. The problem is, healthier, in this case, is still unhealthy.

I submit that it's not peanuts that create the allergic reaction, It's the glucose. Like celiac disease with wheat, peanut allergies operate the same way because they ultimately break down to glucose and then to methylglyoxal, the most glycating substance the body creates from carbs. I contend that it's this substance that causes the allergic reaction. (If it weren't for glucose, the *lac operon* in your genome could recognize all lactose that you consume, but because of this lac operon, your gut bacteria can't recognize the lactose because it sees the glucose. It rejects the lactose making people allergic to lactose, when in all actuality; it's the glucose that's creating the problem.) Where is the warning for glucose? And where's the warning fructose as well for that matter? It glycates, almost as much, as glucose.

Natural Resources Conservation Service (NRCS)

NRCS provides leadership in a partnership effort to help people conserve, maintain and improve our natural resources and environment. (NRCS) is the primary federal agency that works with private landowners to help them conserve, maintain and improve their natural resources. The Agency emphasizes voluntary, science-based conservation; technical assistance; partnerships; incentive-based programs; and cooperative problem-solving at the community level.

This is the agency responsible for the treatment of our environment including the lands and waters that create it. I found that their concern is mostly with conservation and soil health. My concern is in the growing of nonessential grains and feeding them to an unsuspecting society. I included this agency only because it is a small part of this whole complex algorithm. I haven't checked on their relationship with the EPA is though. I'm sure that they would be happy not having to check toxin levels in the soil with the loss of spraying Roundup. I can only imagine the headaches this herbicide has given them (those not owned by Monsanto).

Risk Management Agency (RMA)
RMA helps to ensure that farmers have the financial tools necessary to manage their agricultural risks. RMA provides coverage through the Federal Crop Insurance Corporation which promotes national welfare by improving the economic stability of agriculture. (RMA) promotes, supports, and regulates sound risk management solutions to preserve and strengthen the economic stability of America's agricultural producers by providing crop insurance to American producers, developing and the premium rate, administering premium and expense subsidy, approving and supporting products, and reinsuring companies.

It's a shame crop insurance doesn't cover the damage the crops do to the consumer. Where's that kind of crop insurance? In a keto diet!

Rural Development (RD)

RD helps rural areas to develop and grow by offering Federal assistance that improves quality of life. RD targets communities in need and then empowers them with financial and technical resources. USDA Rural Development is committed to the future of rural communities. Our role is to increase rural residents' economic opportunities and improve their quality of life. Rural Development forges partnerships with rural communities, funding projects that bring housing, community facilities, utilities and other services. We also provide technical assistance and financial backing for rural businesses and cooperatives to create quality jobs in rural areas. Rural Development promotes the President's National Energy Policy and ultimately the nation's energy security by engaging the entrepreneurial spirit of rural America in the development of renewable energy and energy efficiency improvements. Rural Development works with low-income individuals, State, local and Indian tribal governments, as well as private and nonprofit organizations and user-owned cooperatives.
Program and Service Highlights

Business Programs
Community Development Programs
Cooperative Programs
Housing and Community Facilities Programs
Renewable Energy and Energy Efficiency Improvements Program
Rural Utilities Service
Water and Waste Disposal Loan and Grant Program

This agency's concern is the viability of rural communities, probably in an attempt not to allow rural towns to become ghost towns, which is already beginning to happen where industrial farming is taking place. With the new industrial farming that's done today, fewer farmers are living in rural areas to support these rural communities. This is industrial farming according to the Monsanto creed. I shouldn't need to ask you why this is allowed to happen. What will I ask is, what would happen if the grain industry transformed into a healthier industry? It would have to be one that didn't involve polluting the environment with herbicides and pesticides and creating food that is responsible for all modern disease imposed upon modern man. It would have to include a withdrawal from industrial farming, A lack of the need for all the grain we consume would curtail this problem immensely. We need to bring back the small farmer.

Departmental Management (DM)
DM provides central administrative management support to Department officials and coordinates administrative programs and services.

Departmental Management is USDA's central administrative management organization. Departmental Management provides budget and fiscal management, human resource, procurement and information technology support to mission areas so that they can serve customers more effectively and efficiently. Departmental Management manages the Headquarters Complex and provides direct customer service to Washington, D.C. employees.
Program and Service Highlights

Be Prepared - USDA Employee Information Center
Sustainable Operations - USDA Sustainability Efforts
Office of Small and Disadvantaged Business Utilization
TARGET Center
USDA Vendor Outreach Program
Judicial Decisions
Contract Appeal Decisions
Alternative Fuel Vehicle (AFV) Program
Workplace Violence Prevention

If this department's job is to coordinate interdepartmental management and cooperation, is it their responsibility to disseminate the information from the reports in PubMed, PMC, and the FDA with their agency that recommends what should be in our diet? Have they educated the people at MyPlate.gov about the warnings that have been coming from PubMed and PMC about the dangers of what they're recommending everyone to consume on a regular basis? Whole grains are still recommended in every agency and association that has a diet recommendation. Even Myplate.gov and the American Dietary Association and, believe it or not, the American Diabetic Association still recommend whole grains should be a part of a healthy diet. What health grains bring is, by far, counterbalanced by the harm they inflict.

National Appeals Division (NAD)
NAD conducts impartial administrative appeal hearings of adverse program decisions made by USDA and reviews of determinations issued by NAD hearing officers when requested by a party to the appeal. (NAD) is responsible for all administrative appeals arising from program activities of the Farm Service Agency, Risk Management Agency, Natural Resources Conservation Service, Rural Business-Cooperative Development Service, Rural Housing Service, and the Rural Utilities Service.
Program and Service Highlights

Appeal Process
E-Guide to Filing an Appeal
How to Make an FOIA Request
Statutes and Regulations
Search for Decisions

The appeal that I'd like to file would be to appeal the decision to approve grains for human consumption. They're inadequate as animal feed due to all the herbicides and pesticides in them, yet they still recommend them as human food. This is unconscionable.

OFFICES

Office of Advocacy and Outreach (OAO)

The Office of Advocacy and Outreach (OAO) was established by the 2008 Farm bill to improve access to USDA programs and to improve the viability and profitability of small farms and ranches; beginning farmers and ranchers and socially disadvantaged farmers or ranchers. OAO develops and implements plans to coordinate outreach activities and services provided by the Department through working collaboratively with the field base agencies and continually assessing the effectiveness of its outreach programs. Improving the viability and profitability of small and beginning farmers and ranchers Improving access to USDA programs for historically underserved communities Improving agricultural opportunities for farm workers Closing the professional achievement gap by providing opportunities to talented and diverse young people to support the agricultural industry in the 21st century

If it's this department's responsibility to ensure the small farmer's growth, why are they allowing Monsanto to take over all farming in the USA? A healthy food supply cannot be supplied by a monopoly as big as Monsanto. Are they familiar with the contracts Monsanto requires their contracted farmers to sign? Are they familiar with to movement Monsanto is making to control 100% or our food supply? Are they aware of the holdings of the Monsanto execs in the drug industry that used to be owned by Monsanto? I'm sure their breakup did not leave anybody without stock options.

Office of the Assistant Secretary for Civil Rights (OASCR)

OASCR's mission is to facilitate the fair and equitable treatment of USDA customers and employees while ensuring the delivery and enforcement of civil rights programs and activities. ASCR ensures compliance with applicable laws, regulations, and policies for USDA customers and employees regardless of race, color, national origin, sex (including gender identity and expression), religion, age, disability, sexual orientation, marital or familial status, political beliefs, parental status, protected genetic information, or because all or part of an individual's income is derived from any public assistance program. (Not all bases apply to all programs.)

Office of Budget and Program Analysis (OBPA)

OBPA provides centralized coordination and direction for the Department's budget, legislative and regulatory functions. It also provides analysis and evaluation to support the implementation of critical policies. OBPA administers the Department's budgetary functions and develops and presents budget-related matters to Congress, the news media, and the public.

Office of the Assistant Secretary for Civil Rights ensures compliance with applicable laws, regulations, and policies for USDA customers and employees regardless of race, color, national origin, sex (including gender identity and expression), religion, age, disability, sexual orientation, marital or familial status, political beliefs, parental status, protected genetic information, or because all or part of an individual's income is derived from any public assistance program. (Not all bases apply to all programs.)

Program and Service Highlights

Program Discrimination Complaints
Office of the Assistant Secretary for Civil Rights
Early Resolution and Conciliation

If this department is interested in civil rights, then I have a complaint about them right now. My rights have been violated, by this food being imposed upon me, by making sure it's in my baby food, and anything I want to drink (except for plain water), and everything I want to eat. I didn't ask for this but it causes a lot of discomfort for me and everyone else who eats it. All of our rights were violated in serving this food to us without our consent or approval.

Office of the Chief Economist (OCE)
OCE advises the Secretary on the economic situation in agricultural markets and the economic implications of policies and programs affecting American agriculture and rural communities. OCE serves as the focal point for economic intelligence and analysis related to agricultural markets and for risk assessment and cost-benefit analysis related to Departmental regulations affecting food and agriculture. (OCE) advises the Secretary on the economic implications of policies and programs affecting the U.S. food and fiber system and rural areas as well as coordinates, reviews, and approves the Department's commodity and farm sector forecasts.
Program and Service Highlights

World Agricultural Outlook Board (WAOB)
Office of Risk Assessment and Cost-Benefit Analysis
Climate Change Program Office
Sustainable Development
Agricultural Labor Affairs
Office of Energy Policy and New Uses
Weather and Climate

Office of Environmental Markets

If this office is to oversee the offices affecting the food and fiber system, what's happened to the regulation regarding the use of pesticides and herbicides on crops? Is there none?

Office of the Chief Financial Officer (OCFO)
OCFO shapes an environment for USDA officials eliciting the high-quality financial performance needed to make and implement effective policy, management, stewardship, and program decisions. (OCFO) provides financial leadership for USDA, which administers $100 billion of loans as well as significant guarantees and insurance in support of America's farmers and ranchers.
Program and Service Highlights
USDA Budget
USDA Performance and Accountability Report
USDA Strategic Plan
National Finance Center (NFC)
Employee Personal Page
Financial Management Modernization Initiative (FMMI)

I wonder how many loans they've given that have benefited the industrial farming side of this equation. Are they helping to promote this huge industrial farming that's detrimental not only to the environment but to our food supply? How can that be to our benefit?

Office of the Chief Information Officer (OCIO
OCIO has the primary responsibility for the supervision and coordination of the design, acquisition, maintenance, use, and disposal of information technology by USDA agencies. OCIO's strategically acquires and uses information technology resources to improve the quality, timeliness, and cost-effectiveness of USDA services.
Program and Service Highlights
Directives
Enterprise Architecture
Enterprise IT Solutions
Enterprise Network Services
Forms Management
Governance and Strategic Investment (GSI)
Information Collection
IT Capital Planning & Investment Control
IT Security
Quality of Information Guidelines
Records Management
Section 508

This is the IT dept of the USDA. My question for this dept, does their information collection include reports from PubMed and PMC for educational purposes for recommending diets through Myplate.gov?

Office of the Chief Scientist (OCS)
OCS provides scientific leadership to the Department by ensuring that research supported by and scientific advice provided to the Department and its stakeholders is held to the highest standards of intellectual rigor and scientific integrity. It also identifies and prioritizes Department-wide agricultural research, education, and extension needs. (OCS) was established in accordance with the Food, Conservation, and Energy Act of 2008 to provide strategic coordination of the science that informs the Department's and the Federal government's decisions, policies and regulations that impact all aspects of U.S. food and agriculture and related landscapes and communities.
OCS advises USDA's Chief Scientist and the Secretary of Agriculture in the following areas of science:
Agricultural Systems and Technology
Animal Health and Production, and Animal Products
Plant Health and Production, and Plant Products
Renewable Energy, Natural Resources, and Environment
Food Safety, Nutrition, and Health
Agricultural Economics and Rural Communities

Our work supports larger goals of scientific prioritization and coordination across the entire Department through which federal agencies provide Senior Advisors to serve in a detailed capacity within OCS. We identify, prioritize and evaluate Department-wide agricultural research, education, and extension needs. In addition, the Office of the Chief Scientist regularly convenes a USDA Science Council to further facilitate cross-Departmental scientific coordination and collaboration.

That is directly from their website. To me that says that they ensure information gets from one department to another department, yet they seemed to have missed the reports from PubMed and PMC pointing to the damage grains do, especially wheat.

From a PDF document on nutrition, *Executive Summary: National Nutrition Research Roadmap (2016-2021)* I found this paragraph;

For Q3T1 (Assessing Dietary Exposures), ARS scientists recognize there is a strong need for biomarkers of intake, nutrient status, and health, and are working in multiple areas related to this. For example, ARS scientists are studying the association of vitamin K with reduced cardiovascular disease and the amounts and types of dietary fatty acids that influence immunity and inflammation. There is also a need for the development of more objective measures of food intake and physical activity. To that end, scientists are testing electronic capture devices that require no input from the user and can download to databases. I can tell them right now, that fatty acids are very important for immune functions. I've found those studies in my research. If that's what I found, I'm sure that's what they'll find. I also found that all inflammation that exists is because of glucose in the blood. I wonder how long it will be until they realize that all inflammation is influenced by one thing more than anything else? I can tell them with full confidence that glucose influences inflammation more than anything else. I know because I limit my inflammation by limiting my carb intake and nothing else has worked as well. I can also tell them through experience that exercise and dietary reduction of starches, (which they still recommend being 25% of the diet) will go further than any vitamin. I wonder how long it will take this chief scientist to realize that glycation is at the root of all inflammation and that glucose is at the root of all glycation. It doesn't take any kind of a scientist to see that if you removed the glucose from the equation, the product of the equation couldn't exist. The product in this equation is all the diseases created by inflammation.

Office of Communications (OC)
OC is USDA's central source of public information. The office provides centralized information services using the latest, most effective and efficient technology and standards for communication. It also provides the leadership, coordination, expertise, and counsel needed to develop the strategies, products, and services that are used to describe USDA initiatives, programs, and functions to the public. (OC) provides leadership, expertise, counsel, and coordination for the development of communications strategies which are vital to the overall formulation, awareness, and acceptance of USDA programs and policies, and serves as the principal USDA contact point for the dissemination of consistent, timely information.
Program and Service Highlights
Creative Media and Broadcast Center
Brand, Events, Exhibits, and Editorial Review
Digital Communications
Photography Services
Printing Services
Radio News

The dissemination of consistent, timely information, is what this office's responsibility is, yet I've not heard anything from them about the information from over 11,750 studies recording the dangers of glycation, which is the result of glucose interference with your body's normal processes. With studies showing this glycation going back over 30 years (about as old as GMO seeds), why hasn't any of this *"timely information"* been *disseminated* for *30 years*? Is this due to the Monsanto influence? If any agency is not fulfilling their responsibilities to keep the public safe from their own food, it's this one. They have access to the same studies that I and thousands of others do, yet they still choose to ignore them. They still choose to recommend that this poisonous food be a part of your diet. Why?

Office of Congressional Relations (OCR)

OCR serves as the USDA's liaison with Congress. OCR works closely with members and staffs of various House and Senate Committees to communicate the USDA's legislative agenda and budget proposals. (OCR) serves as the Department's liaison with Members of Congress and their staffs. OCR works closely with members and staffs of various House and Senate Committees including the House Agriculture Committee and the Senate Committee on Agriculture, Nutrition, and Forestry to communicate USDA's legislative agenda and budget proposals. Within OCR is the Office of External and Intergovernmental Affairs (EIA) which serves as the liaison to elected and appointed officials of State, county, local, and Tribal governments. The office also serves as a liaison to USDA stakeholders.

My question to this office, have your alerted Congress of the dangers of these grains and the consequences they bring to the human physiology when consumed? Are you afraid of laws being passed that might outlaw some of this insanity? The insanity that I refer to is the insanity of buying into this glucose ruse, orchestrated by one of the most unscrupulous companies to ever conduct business. Is this the office responsible for keeping this information hidden from our lawmakers' eyes? Is this the office that should be held accountable for our current state of public health? The state of our current public health is obese and diabetic, leading to carcinogenic and atherosclerotic, all because of the inflammatory nature of glycation.

If I can learn this myself and I have a good deal of brain damage inhibiting my learning ability, why can't this office learn this to alert our Congress of this problem? The problem exists only for the consumer, as it's a boom for Monsanto and its industries. Why would they want to control this? For them, this is good business. This is what attracts stockholders.

Office of Ethics (OE)

The Office of Ethics (OE) is the centralized office responsible for coordinating and implementing USDA's Ethics program throughout the Department. OE provides ethics services to employees at all levels of USDA concerning advice and training about compliance with ethics laws and regulations, including the conflict of interest and impartiality rules, as well as the rules governing political activity by Federal employees.

A visit to this office's site brought me to a page that showed me;

THE STOCK ACT

On April 4, 2012, the President signed the Stop Trading on Congressional Knowledge Act or STOCK Act (S. 2038), which amended the Ethics in Government Act of 1978 (5 U.S.C. App. § 101 et seq.) The Act has several different provisions, some of which are effective immediately, some which become effective 90 days after enactment, some which become effective on August 31, 2012, and some which do not become effective until 18 months after enactment. *The following compendium of ethics laws, regulations and guidelines govern Executive Branch employees' conduct, including USDA employees. The Department promulgated its own supplemental ethics regulation (5 CFR Part 8301) in 2006 to augment the Office of Government Ethics' Standards of Ethical Conduct. The Department's ethics regulation and other selected ethics laws and regulations are accessible from this page for ready reference (click on "General Ethics Laws and Regulations" below).*

Overviews
Ethics Issuances
General Ethics Laws and Regulations
USDA Supplemental Ethics Regulations 🗗

Financial Disclosure
Fundraising & the CFC
Gifts
Holiday Guidance for Federal Personnel
Letters of Support, Recommendation, Collaboration, etc.
Lobbying
Non-Federal Organizations
Outside Employment
Political Activity
Post Employment and Seeking Employment
Procurement Integrity 🗗
Special Government Employees (SGEs)
STOCK Act
Travel & Non-Federal Assistance

I wonder what their ethic regulations say about recommending poisonous food to remain in our diet when there is proof of this food's glycative effects in over 10,000 studies in PubMed and PMC. What do their ethics say about falsifying information disseminated to the public? The still claim that whole grains are safe to eat.

Office of Environmental Markets (OEM)
OEM supports the development of emerging markets for carbon, water quality, wetlands, and biodiversity. (OEM) provides leadership in the development of emerging markets for carbon, water quality, wetlands, and biodiversity. OEM is building national environmental market infrastructure,

supporting regional market innovation, and fostering collaboration around market-based conservation within USDA and across the federal government.

I wonder if this environmental market infrastructure includes more fields of these killing field grains? If so, they may want to re-assess their goals, if they intend to protect the public and the environment.

Office of the Executive Secretariat (OES)
OES ensures that all Department officials are included in the correspondence drafting and policy-making process through a managed clearance and control system. Keeping policy officials informed of executive documents enhances the Secretary's ability to review sound and thought out policy recommendations before making final decisions. (OES) ensures that all Department officials are included in the correspondence drafting and policy-making process through a managed clearance and control system. Keeping policy officials informed of executive documents enhances the Secretary's ability to review sound and thought out policy recommendations before making final decisions. Did this office miss the memo on glycation; its causes and effects? Do they need another one? Is it their responsibility that so few know about this? Are these the people we should hold accountable?

Faith-Based and Neighborhood Partnerships (FBNP)
USDA has a long historyy of working with faith-based and communityy organizations to help those in need, by providing federal assistance through domestic nutrition assistance programs, international food aid, rural development opportunities, and natural resource conservation.

This is the office that coordinates churches food banks to assist the needy. Every church I've been to has had one, and they all give out plenty of bread, the deadliest of foods that we can give anyone. This condemns these poor unsuspecting souls to lives of poor health and continued medication. Our food supply is inundated with this vile product, only because it's the primary bringer of people to medication, medication for pain.

Office of the Inspector General (OIG)
OIG investigates allegations of crime against the Department's program and promotes the economy and efficiency of its operations. (OGC) is an independent legal agency that provides legal advice and services to the Secretary of Agriculture and to all other officials and agencies of the Department with respect to all USDA programs and activities.

There were 50,000 food safety inspections in 1972. That was reduced to just over 9,000 in 2008. If there were only 9000 in 2008, reduced from 50,000 in 1972, when the threat level was much lower, the FDA is only succeeding at failing us on an unprecedented basis. I'm sure this is due to funding cutbacks from the government but I'm also sure it involves something related to departmental offices being run by corporate management brought in from corporations they're supposed to regulate, proving once again (unfortunately) the bottom line is what wins here and the bottom line is greed.

If the USDA and the FDA can allow a food this dangerous through its monitoring, I'm afraid to even think about what else has snuck through? The beef industry has already displayed their contempt for regulation through the mass production of beef that their industry is responsible for, especially in the last 30 years.

Office of the General Counsel (OGC)
The Office of the General Counsel (OGC) is an independent legal agency that provides legal advice and services to the Secretary of Agriculture and to all other officials and agencies of the Department with respect to all USDA programs and activities.

I wonder how many lawsuits this agency is going to have to fight for advising the public to eat food that's as dangerous as whole grains. Myplate.gov still has them at 25% of our diet. Why?

Office of Tribal Relations (OTR)
The Office of Tribal Relations is located in the Office of the Secretary and is responsible for government-to-government relations between USDA and tribal governments.

I can only empathize with this office as they have to see that this garbage is provided to tribal governments as well as the public in general.
I listed all of their offices and agencies for a reason. I wanted to show you the vastness of this department. It's huge. It has to be huge to protect our food supply. As big as it is, it's not doing that. It's not doing its job. It's been hijacked by the industry that it's supposed to control. The proof lies in the extent of which disease exists today.

With all of these agencies and offices, I'm sure it's quite difficult to keep all this information straight for the public to fully understand what this agency is allowing to "fall through the cracks", as in allowing grains and sugar to be recommended food for everyone to eat, sometimes even those who have celiac disease. What this agency doesn't understand is that everyone has an intolerance to the gluten that comes in grains. It's estimated that 95% of the population have some sort of intolerance to the gliadin and gluten found in most cereal grains, especially wheat, barley, and rye.

I've already contacted the **Center for Nutrition Policy and Promotion0**

(CNPP) to ask them why they still recommend including grains in the diet. They've come to their senses when it comes to sugar, why can't they, with grains, they're just as deadly as sugar, if not more so? The agency above is responsible for recommending our diet at My Plate and I've already asked them why they still recommend a food that can cause as much damage is this food does. I'm waiting for their reply.

There is absolutely no reason for these foods to still be recommended except for the fact that to decrease the consumption of this food would irreparably harm Monsanto and the farming industry that they control. And they control a huge portion of it.

The infiltration of their old execs and lobbyists into the offices of the FDA and the USDA is evidence indicating their complicity in the matter. With their old personnel working the offices and agencies of the USDA and the FDA, they've cleared a pathway to their full control over what goes on your table. This in return gives them control over the meds you'll be buying from them in the near future.

I noticed that there is no agency or office to review and disseminate the information in these research studies showing the damaging effects of the food they're recommending for us to eat. There's supposed to be one, but there isn't.

How do they make recommendations on what foods are good for you to eat, when you're ignoring all the studies that say otherwise? They rely on Monsanto to tell them what's healthy and what isn't. Is that a source you would trust? I hope so because you trust them with every bagel you put in your mouth.

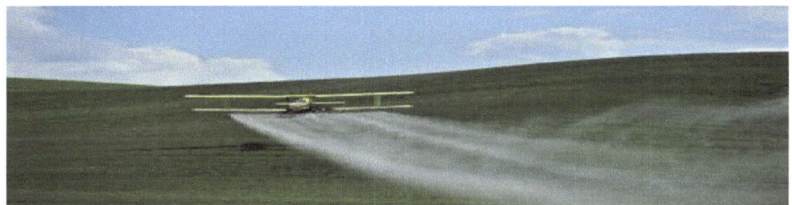

Monsanto's Field of disease and discomfort

CHAPTER 10

INDUSTRY'S INFLUENCE IN THE EXPANSION OF CARB PRODUCTION

It would be nice if money weren't the primary motivating factor in business. It would be nice if the health and welfare of every individual human being were the primary motivating factors in business. But it's not. That is why this chapter may be the hardest one to construct. It not only involves corporate America, it involves a major portion of all industry, both big and small, even down to the mom and pop stores in small town, America, and that's what makes this chapter so hard to write.

The problem is that this problem invades the very core of our society, our sustenance. This is what we all work for. Our primary goal, for our families, (after finding shelter) is to put food on the table. And this is where the problem begins. Everyone has to eat. This makes everyone, who's hungry, susceptible to outside influences, to quench those hunger pangs.

The food industry understands this. They've done numerous studies on it. Their research has told them how, when, where, and to whom to market their products to. All so they can increase their profits. Their only interest, though, is to please their stockholders, they not interested in their customer's health (except for a few in the health industry), and so everything they do, is done for the bottom line, profit. Because of this shortsightedness, and not looking that far into the future, they disregard for the health of their customers is unimportant to them. They only want your money.

These products kill because of the sugar they contain, we all know that. But the problem here is, that they don't kill immediately, so they're legal. Their death sentence takes a lot longer. It's a lot more painful. It's a lot more expensive. It's a lot more emotionally draining. Many times it's more violent. It's definitely, nothing anyone should have to experience, yet the addiction, keeps anyone who's on this diet remain on this diet, voluntarily. Only those strong enough can break the cycle of addiction. But the beauty of breaking it is this, it doesn't take that long, as long as you can abstain from its lure. It only takes a week or two, for the average addict. Heavier, more addicted people might take another month or two. It's even quicker if you fast.

Bringing the food industry to an understanding, that they are sacrificing tomorrow's customers for today's profits, may help in curbing corporate influence, but is it enough to change the behavior of all corporate America? I don't know. The amount of change that would have to occur is enormous because the industry is enormous. How do you change an industry this enormous? With the pharmaceutical industry's interest at hand, I don't see the situation getting any better any time soon. The only way I know how to is to let them know that what they're doing is not acceptable by a long shot. We must let this industry that what they're doing is irreprehensible and not go on any longer.

Unfortunately, profit doesn't have a soul. It has no moral values. And it's the moral values that make us a society. Without them, we'd have no laws or regulations to keep people from stepping on other people's toes. This begs the question, what role does profit play in a civilized culture. Most of us know that profit = money. Most of us also know that a civilization needs money to conduct commerce, so everyone within that civilization can trade their goods and services. It's this trade, that's at the core of civilization. People came together in primitive times for protection, and this, in turn, started us trading our possessions and food. And thus, the beginning of commerce, the engine that keeps our society, culture, and civilization growing.

If it's the desire of money, that's at the root of all evil, does that make all of corporate America evil, because of their desire to improve their profits? Some would say so, simply because of the lack of responsibility corporate America takes for their actions when they harm others. Others would say, it's survival. In all actuality, it's both. The desire for profit and power is what drives almost all of corporate America. It's my opinion, that this is where corporate America is failing society.

Because they have to fulfill stockholders wishes to make more money, they are obligated to do so. Doing anything else would not be considered profitable and it wouldn't keep the stockholders happy. The company would lose the investment of their stockholders and this, in turn, would strongly disable their ability to conduct business and therein threaten the existence of the company. Profit is important. It's one of the biggest, if not the biggest motivating factors in our society.

We, in the United States, have always used our freedoms, to bolster our efforts to increase our profits. It's this freedom, that's built the strongest empire in history. The problem is this when you consider freedom and what it brings us, you have to look at the other side of the coin, that freedom is on. The other side of this freedom coin, that's tossed around so much (mostly politically), is responsibility. You can't have true freedom without responsibility. The responsibility side of the coin, says, that you must take responsibility for the freedoms you enjoy, especially when those freedoms inflict harm on another human being. You can't have true freedom without this responsibility.

Without the responsibility, what do you have? A society without control. When any one person, group, or company isn't fully responsible for enjoying their freedoms, where does the freedom exist for all parties? In that sense then, where does it exist for anyone? It doesn't when one does harm to any other person or group. This is where the problem lies. Only one person's freedom was expressed. The person on whom this expression of freedom was committed, wasn't allowed to express their own freedom because they were subjected to the freedoms of the other. Is this really true freedom? I submit, that it isn't, it's not true freedom at all. At best, it's pseudo-freedom and it sounds a lot like slavery.

It's how our system, works, and because our Supreme Court thinks that corporations are the same as people, they deserve the same rights and freedoms as any single individual human being. Do corporations have the same morals as most human beings? Yet, they're allowed a lot more freedom, simply because, they have the money to do so.

Here's the worst part of this, equation. It's because of your addiction. It's your money they use. You give it to them, freely, every time you buy their products. At least you think you do. What you think is your own choice, to purchase what you think is healthy food, is actually you succumbing to their desire. You are slaves to their wishes, every time you bag their groceries…and later on years down the road, their drugs.

This is a trap, that I refuse to fall into. I can only thank Dr. Perlmutter, Dr. Davis, and Dr. Amen, for setting me on the path that brought me to this point, and this book, (I don't mention Dr. Amen anywhere in any of my articles, except right here. The reason I mention him here, is because he's the one who basically started me on this journey.)

Carbohydrates are a food of emotion. It's how they make you fat. They control your emotions. They'll continue to control your emotions until you give them up and thus in doing so, control them. Nothing controls me. What do you let control you?

Industry Concerns of Dispelling Wheat and Grains

What moves America forward or backward, more than anything else, is corporate advancement or hindrance. Hence the control of corporations in America is what drives this advancement or decline, and proliferation of a grain-based diet has benefitted the grain industry and the drug industry but it has devastated our health. This to me is an unconscionable act and it must change if we're to save our society.

If any major change is to occur within the realms of modern society, it must be done, on a corporate level. This brings us to the dilemma of how to change the behavior of millions of people, all who are addicted to these substances and worse yet addicted to what corporate America tells them to do. They tell them how to think, how to eat, what to drink, primarily what they should be eating and drinking. This puts them in control of the amount of sugar we consume, which in turn, controls our emotions, to put us 'under their spell', so to speak. They're never going to want to give that up. That's something that we have to take back. and that's why the site URL is SAVEOURDIGNITY.ORG. In order to affect, changes in the food industry, primarily the grain industry, you need to make corporate America know, that you're tired of this abuse and don't want to lose your dignity. The dignity that Alzheimer's disease robs you of, that heart disease takes and that cancer cancels out. It's time to cure corporate America of its addiction to hunger.

It must be incorporated into this network of our society that change must happen. The problem therein lies, this industry is huge. It's comprised of, probably more companies, than any other industry, in the world, as food is the most important commodity that's marketed worldwide. The number of companies in this industry is almost unimaginable. So how do we change the behavior of this much of our society? It can't be done overnight. It's going to take the efforts of everyone in society, to make a change, this grandiose, which means it's going to take a while. Corporate industry, the food industry primarily, must confront the dangers, that they are imposing the entire world, by continuing to grow, manufacture, market, advertise and sell this devastating food that causes so many illnesses and diseases. They must understand that killing their customers, is not a solid business plan. Even the ones addicted to their treatments will eventually expire sooner, rather than later. Where's the sense in it?

I realize that many of the crop seed companies, (Monsanto, Dupont, Syngenta, Land O' Lakes, Bayer and many other overseas), have had a lot of the money tied up in pharmaceuticals, as well as manufacturing the crop seed, (much of it genetically modified to withstand their chemical herbicides and pesticides). Even though many of those companies liquidated their investments in the pharmaceutical side of the industry, many of these companies still have ties to each other, which begs the question, were cover-ups initiated to help hide these facts? It conjures, in my mind, the question of how threatened did they feel if any of this information was released to the public? Are these valid arguments? I think so. And I think they deserve further investigation. This endeavor is where it gets interesting. With corporate America in so much control of how our society functions, it's occurred to me that nothing is going to happen, until corporate America, the food industry and pharmaceutical industry, in general, must change their behavior, They must discontinue the marketing and advertising of these products, so as to not persuade the public that they need to continue to eat this garbage. The question arises, how do you make a company cut its own throat. If anything were to interrupt the flow of their finances, how long can they stay in business? This brings us to the core of what we need to work toward, to change, and changing it, may result in much of this industry re-assessing their goals of placing human health at risk for the sake of profits.

The soft drink industry, for example, they're probably the most guilty of any, for slipping this dangerous food into our diet, by loading up their drinks with high-fructose corn syrup, sugar, Aspartame, Cyclamate, Saccharin, Sucralose, Acesulfame potassium, malt syrup, Lead acetate, any many others that I have trouble pronouncing, like maltodextrin, maltitol, maltotriose, Icodextrin, and too many forms of oligosaccharides to list here. To find them all, you need to refer to every food label on every can of soft drink, that's on the market. Convincing the beverage industry of finding other sources of sweeteners is already beginning to take place. A lot of manufacturers are starting to offer drinks sweetened with Stevia, a completely natural, non-caloric sweetener, that's super concentrated when it's offered in powdered form. My wish is for the transformation of all sweetened drinks to Stevia instead of the high sugar sweeteners, like all of those listed above. Can you imagine what this would do, to get this dangerous substance out of our diet? I can. You can visit my dream page in my first book.

So how do we replace the lost business and everything else that goes along with it, the jobs and careers, the investment of millions of Americans, who've all invested in these companies(through their IRA'S, Keoghs, investment funds, etc)? How do we take away all of that? The problem is, you can't, and that's where the problem of dispelling this problem lies. You have to replace what you take away, with healthier options. If it's healthier for the body, it's healthier for business and corporate America. My contention is that business or corporate America, and the health of the individual run hand in hand. Why then, does the crop seed industry continue in its deadly crusade to feed us injurious products with their glyphosate laden grains? I guess when you control an industry that depends on how sick you can make the population along with the industry that supplies them with those very foods to make you sick it becomes the ultimate con game. I was once told "the ideal con is the one you don't see before it hits you and you don't know what's hitting you, while it's hitting you. This is the definition of the perfect con. It's completely legal yet deadly for the victim.

Sherri always told me to

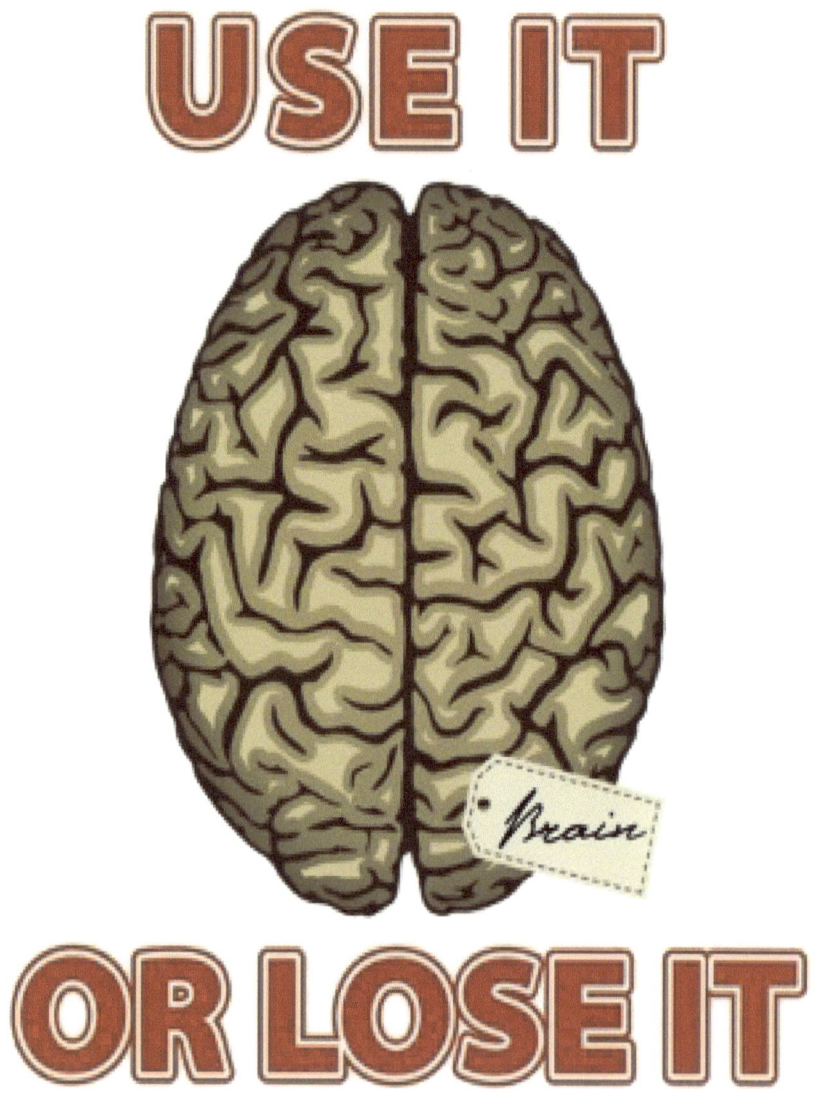

ABOUT THE AUTHOR

3 years ago after suffering from chronic severe pain for 20 years and taking opioid and anti-depressant medication for the pain, I had to endure 16 of those years, I decided something had to change. On top of the drugs I was taking for pain, I was taking drugs to counteract the side effects of the opioids and anti-depressants and they weren't killing the pain. The pain was always there, I was overweight and constipated most of the time, from the drugs I was taking and I had had enough, I'd tried every form of pain relief that I could find, from laser therapy for 15 treatments, to acupuncture 2-3 times a week for years at a time, (that was expensive) to TENS treatments to SCENAR therapy to massage therapy to pain blocks (after I had 5 treatments in 5 months, the doctor refused to inject me again, saying that he'd already injected me with too many steroids), yet the blocks worked for about 30 days, then quit, so I had to go back for another. For 4 years I carried an internal nerve stimulator that I'm sure to cost the insurance plenty of money. That thing worked excellently to mask the pain, but it didn't kill it. The pain was always there under the stimulation however the stimulation masked the pain really well. I used that device so much I wore it out after a couple years and had to have it replaced. The SCENAR is the only device that killed the pain but it didn't last much more than one day. That's why I needed a change, so I changed the last thing I could think of changing, my diet. I quit eating bread. Two weeks later and 10 lbs lighter, magic started to happen. Even though It was the toughest thing I've ever had to accomplish, I quit. I ate no more bread, pasta, crackers, tortillas and potato chips and cut way back on the sodas. Actually, I replaced those with juices, which were better at the time, but I've since quit those also. In the last three years, I've modified my diet to a completely ketogenic diet, concentrating my diet on dairy products (mostly milk). I keep my weight at 10 lbs below my prescribed weight and without eating much of anything all day long, I don't get hungry and I don't get sick. That is the largest blessing of a ketogenic diet. Because I can't afford the treatments and the drugs, I stay on my ketogenic diet.

The bonus I get from staying on my keto diet is multiple, no inflammation, less pain and believe it or not, fewer mosquito bites. Due to the lack of glucose flowing through my blood, mosquitoes can't smell it on my breath. They smell acetone on my breath, which means that I don't have glucose in my body. I like that benefit. I can remember times when I had over 70 mosquito bites on my body at any one time. Argh, was that itchy. It's so nice to not have to deal with that now. No glucose was all it took. That in itself is as good a reason as any, to give up your addiction.

www.ingramcontent.com/pod-product-compliance
Lightning Source LLC
Chambersburg PA
CBHW040903180526
45159CB00010BA/2910